The Pilates Companion

Lyn O'Neill

in collaboration with the Scott Studio

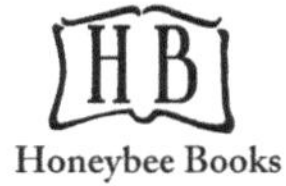

Honeybee Books

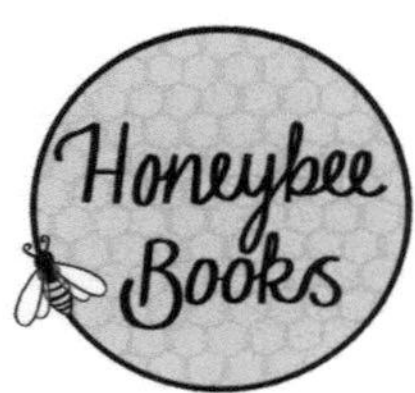

Published by Honeybee Books, Dorset
www.honeybeebooks.co.uk

Text and Images Copyright © Lyn O'Neill 2018

The right of Lyn O'Neill to be identified as the author of this work has been asserted by her in accordance with the Copyright, Designs and Patents Act 1988.

No part of this book may be reproduced in any form or by any electronic or mechanical means including information storage and retrieval systems without permission in writing from the author.

Printed in the UK using paper from sustainable sources

ISBN: 978-1-910616-81-9

This book is not intended as a substitute for the medical advice of physicians. The reader should regularly consult a physician in matters relating to his/her health. Before practicing the skills described in this book consult a doctor to ensure you are ready to begin exercises, and do not take risks beyond your level of experience, aptitude, training, or comfort level.

The information in this book is meant to supplement, not replace, an accredited Pilates training. Like any sport Pilates poses some inherent risk. The author and publisher advise readers to take full responsibility for their safety and know their limits.

Contents

The Pilates Companion is a wonderful resource for Pilates enthusiasts and instructors at any level. The illustrations beautifully convey complex information in a useful and easily absorbed way. Lyn presents Pilates in a way anyone can use. New students will find her explanations easy to understand and embody while experienced practitioners and teachers will be delighted by the lively way the information is presented. I recommend this book to anyone looking to understand the practice of Pilates.

Nora St. John, M.S., PMA-CPT

Education Program Director | Balanced Body Inc, Sacramento, USA.

Foreword

When The Scott Studio opened in 1996, I hoped people who didn't live in London might embrace Pilates even if they were not intending to become professional dancers and hadn't got a back problem. Fortunately, as it turns out, Pilates thrives outside an urban environment: it seems farmers, butchers, dressage riders and great-grandfathers find it helps them go about their business, just as much as ballerinas going about theirs.

In the early days before I eventually started my Teacher Training Programme in Somerset, tutorials were mostly about the two D's: Demonstrate and Do. A lot of stick people were drawn (there was even a tutorial on it), and a lot of paper covered with highlighter pen and exercise hieroglyphics, by diligent students attempting to capture the elusive grammar of Pilates. Despite the bloom of technology and the ease of recording electronically, some things still didn't make it into the download, most notably the presence of the teacher, a guide to the perplexed student wrestling with the anatomy ("the ischial-tube-y what?"), confused by the language ("what do you mean: smile with your hips?") and struggling to remember ("I wrote that you breathe *in* on the leg bit and *out* when you roll over your feet"). A lot of the note taking, including my own, did not make much sense when you came back to it, and whilst the many books on Pilates were good at showing what exercises should look like, the subtleties of intention and feeling, which are fundamental to Pilates, seemed resistant to being recorded.

The first time I caught sight of one of Lyn's drawings in a tutorial was a revelation: here was Pilates on paper, presented in a way that did make sense. The genius of what Lyn has managed to do in The Pilates Companion is to restore the parts that can go missing outside as well as inside a Pilates class: explanations that give context to the (sometimes strange) exercise instructions, images that cut through the tangle of words, technical information that enables self-practice without the patient hand and fierce eye of a teacher looking on.

This book won't replace a good teacher and isn't intended to. However, and as its name suggests, it will make a good companion: one that will guide you expertly, and with a lively sense of wit and humour, through the mystery, the challenge and the s-l-o-w (sometimes called 'boring') of Pilates. If it succeeds in making this extraordinary exercise method accessible to more people, The Pilates Companion, like the small studio in Somerset where it began, will be doing something right.

Suzanne Scott, The Scott Studio, Somerset, England.

November 2017.

Introduction

I'm guessing that if you pick up this book you may already do Pilates and know that it is a good way to exercise, in order to increase flexibility and strengthen the body.

Are you someone who tries to remember an exercise you have been taught but by the end of the class you have forgotten it? You may be someone who has been advised to strengthen your back muscles or your abdominals. Perhaps you are a teacher, physiotherapist or osteopath looking for safe exercises to recommend to your clients.

Even if you have never done it before, the book is for any of you, designed to accompany you on your Pilates journey.

It is intended as an addition to your regular Pilates classes and NOT as a substitute for a teacher. The exercises originate from what is known as the progressed Pilates repertoire and are modified from Joseph Pilates original exercises that appear in full at the end of the book.

I hope you enjoy this irreverent disclosure of my day to day teaching world.

Lyn O'Neill

Section Guide

Section 1

Getting Started

Section 1 gives some insight into how Pilates works with a short introduction to human anatomy and physiology.

Section II

The Essentials

Now it is time to roll out your mat and make yourself comfortable. Even doing ten minutes of Pilates exercise a day will make big difference to your body and keep away those niggling aches and pains. Pick and mix or start with the exercises marked 1 and work your way to 3 and 4.

We start with the basic 'bread and butter' exercises taught in a level 1 and 2 Pilates class. The Essential exercises will be repeated throughout your Pilates journey so it is well worth mastering them.

Numbered strips 1 to 4 indicate the degree of difficulty: Level 1 incorporates beginner to progressed beginner levels. Level 2 progresses you out of being a beginner. Level 3 progresses you into Intermediate exercises. Level 4 exercises are more challenging, demanding better technique.

Work through the strips marked 1 on different pages. Start putting them together to make your own Pilates class. Add the next level and then the final ones.

If you feel any pain or discomfort doing the exercises be sure to drop back a level until you are stronger.

Section III

Pushing On

Try adding some of these higher level exercises to your workout. Be sensible and stop if anything hurts. The exercises get more strenuous, similar to a level 3 Pilates class. Many form part of Joseph Pilates' original repertoire listed in the final chapter.

Section IV

A Workout a Day

This chapter honours the teaching of my fellow teachers and their creativity. Follow each class from beginning to end. You will be introduced to some small items of Pilates equipment such as balls, therabands, yoga bricks and foam rollers that will liven up your practice.

Troubleshooting

Which exercises are safe for me?

Most of the exercises can be done by any healthy person, but as teachers we would always recommend getting advice from your doctor if you are in any doubt about your ability to exercise.

However there are some exercises that should be avoided by certain individuals.

Exercise advice given below is generally considered correct, but please consult your doctor for confirmation before beginning exercise.

Osteoporosis:

Some exercises need to be avoided by those suffering from Osteoporosis, however there are many exercises that are safe to do.

Safe exercises are:

Quadruped
All Butts
The Bridge
Sideways
Arch Your Back to a Healthy Spine
Rotate Your Spine (Level 1 & 2 only)
Leg Circles (Level 1 & 2 only)
Press the Ground Away (Avoid side plank)

Pregnancy

1st Trimester: your usual exercise programme should be safe to do

2nd Trimester: Safe Exercises are:

Quadruped
All Butts
Sideways (Avoid lying on your side for too long)
Rotate Your Spine (Level 1 only)
Sidebend with Strength (Level 1 & 2)
Press the Ground Away (Level 1)

3rd Trimester: same as 2nd Trimester but again avoid lying on your side for too long. Add more kneeling and standing postures or modify your work by sitting on a Gym ball. (Look at Carla's workout for Gym ball exercises p61 and Liz for standing routines p 57).

No loaded abdominal work is recommended after the first trimester.

Obesity

If you have been diagnosed as being clinically obese, follow the guidelines for the Pregnancy second Trimester workout until you have reduced your weight. Then start with the Level 1 exercises.

Section 1

Getting Started

It's the MIND itself which shapes the BODY

Joseph Pilates

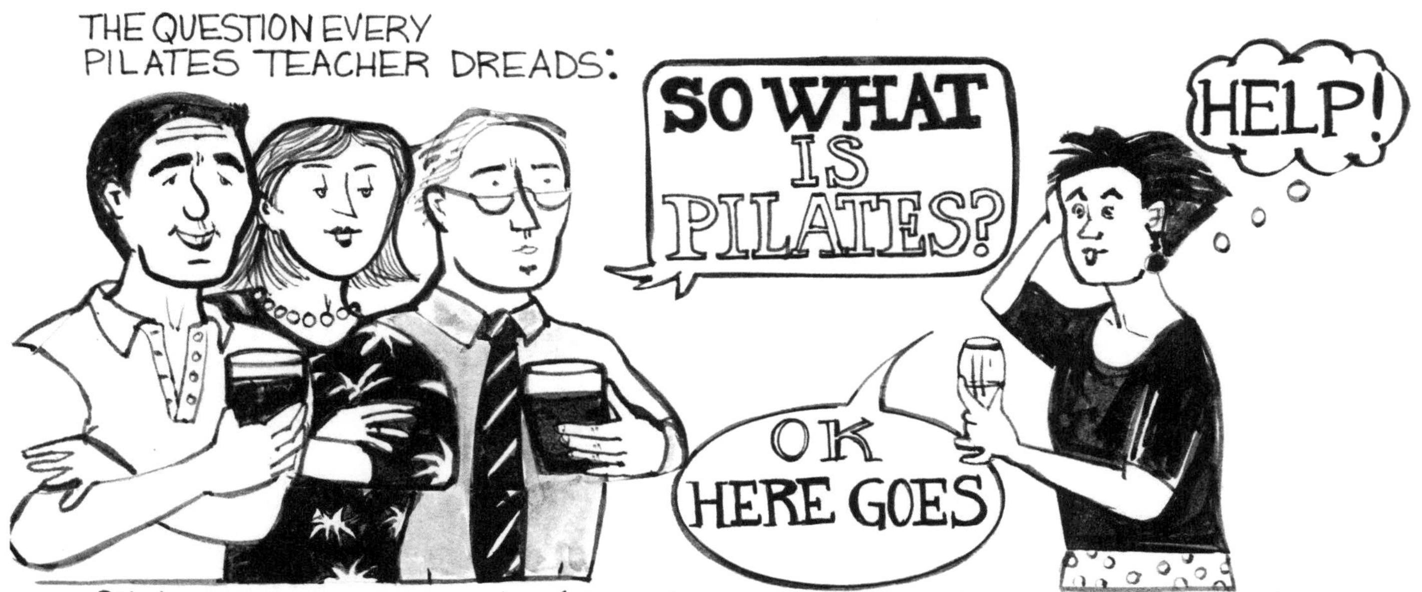

Pilates is an exercise method based on evidence that long term physical fitness can only be sustained if muscle strength includes a strong core & correct posture. This means joints & muscles need to be properly aligned to enable joints to move freely becoming less prone to injury. Every Pilates exercise is very precise, aiming to improve strength & flexibility.

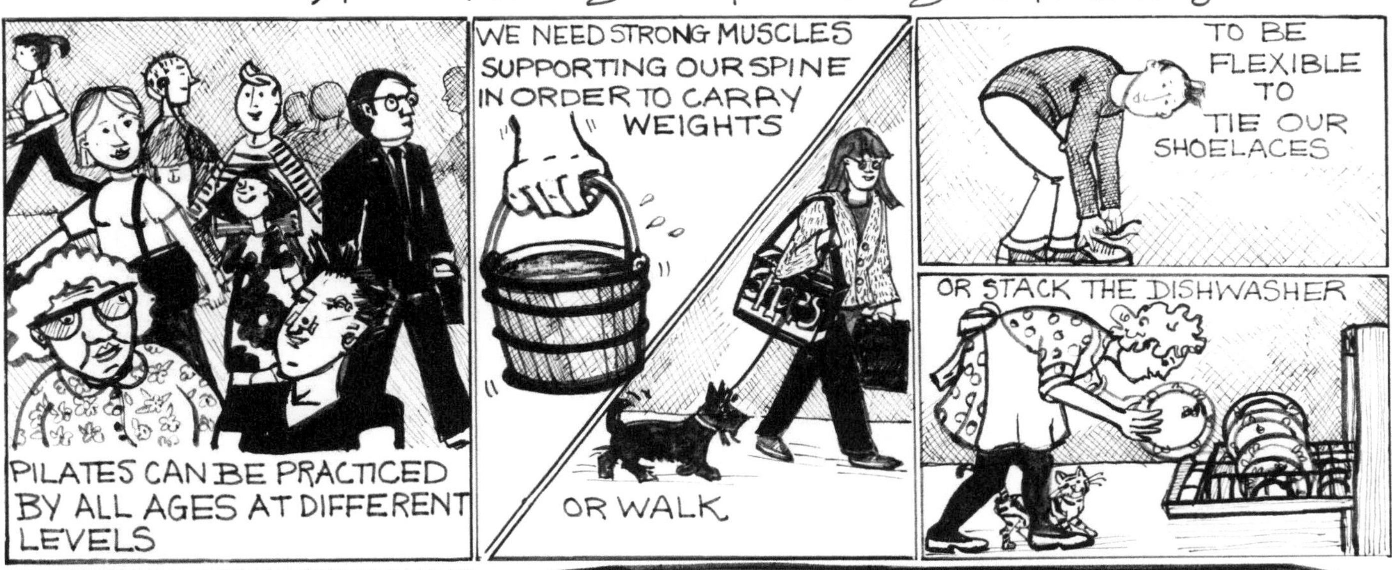

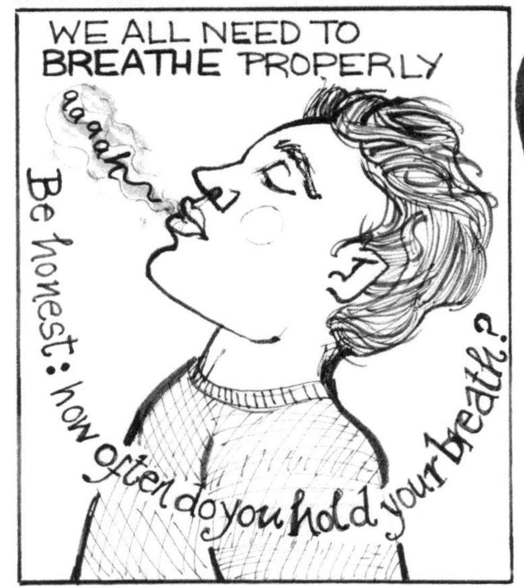

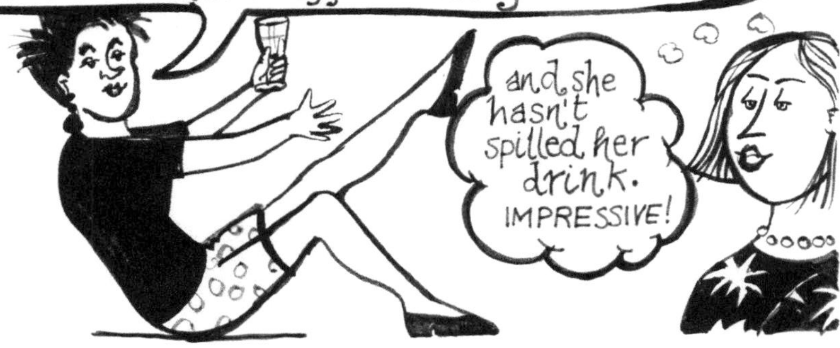

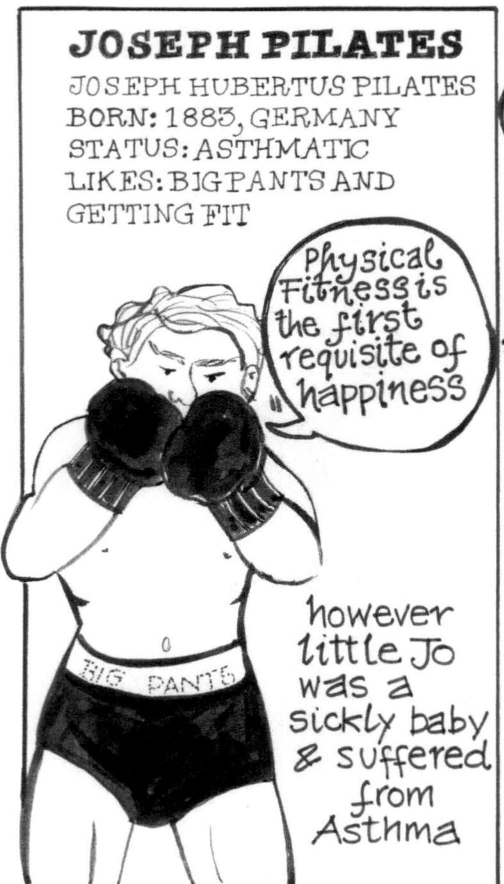

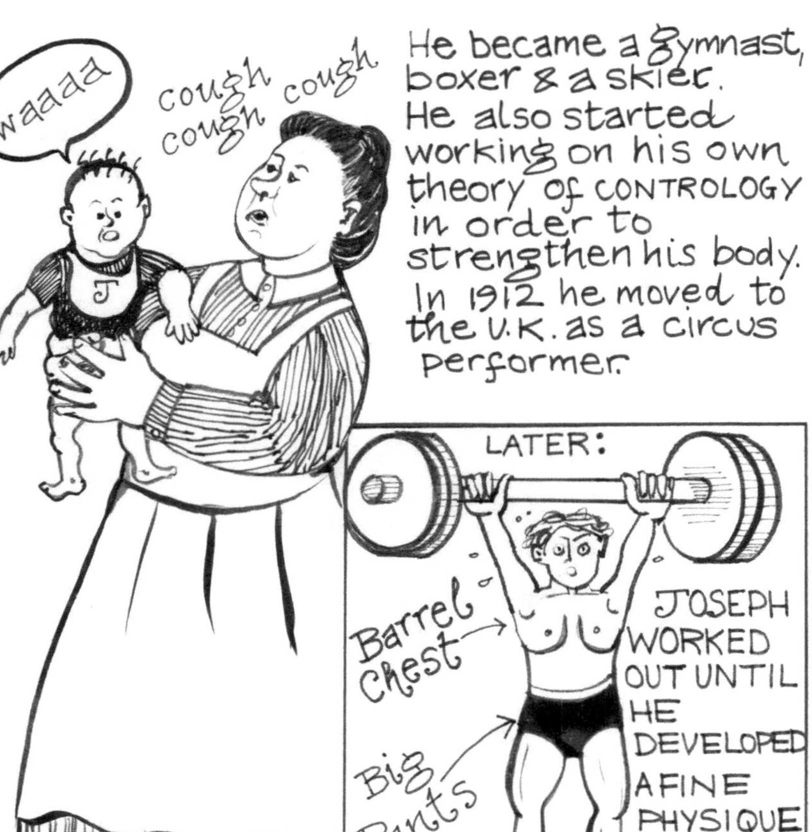

At the outbreak of World War I Jo was interned on the Isle of Man. He became a hospital orderly & helped to rehabilitate injured servicemen by attaching springs to their sick beds & supervising them until they recovered.

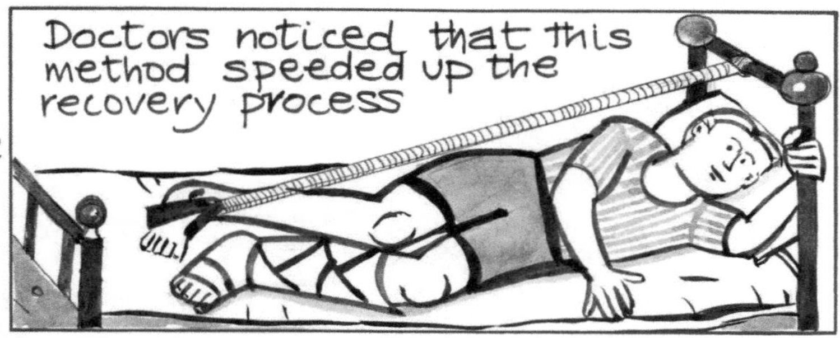

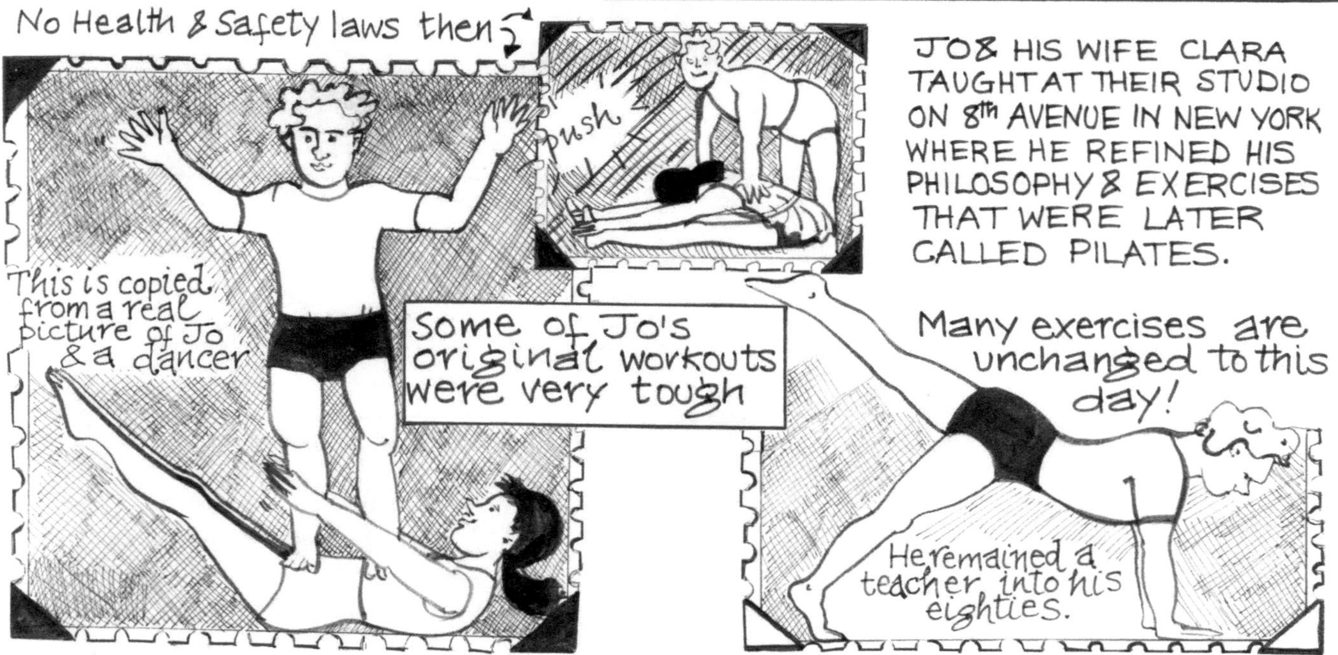

JO USED HIS EXPERIENCE IN INTERNMENT TO BUILD SPRING LOADED EQUIPMENT THAT IS STILL USED IN PILATES STUDIOS NOWADAYS. THE MACHINES ALL HAVE STRANGE NAMES!

The CADILLAC is the most similar to the hospital bed in the previous picture. It looks a bit like a giant bedstead with lots of springs attached to it. You can lie on your back, sides, front or kneel or sit or stand.

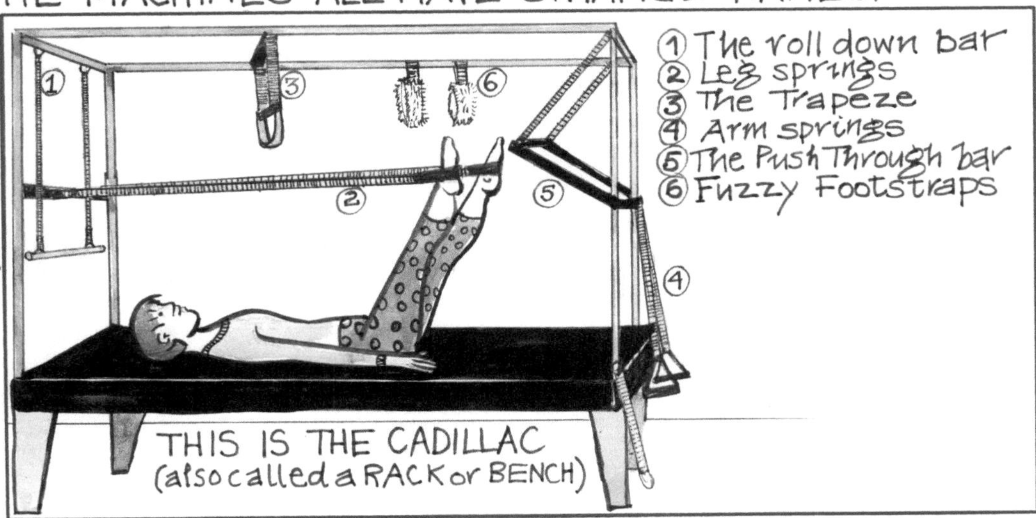

THIS IS THE CADILLAC (also called a RACK or BENCH)

EACH MACHINE HAS A UNIQUE WAY OF WORKING THE DIFFERENT PARTS OF THE BODY. THE SPRINGS WILL WORK THE ARM OR LEG MUSCLES BUT ENCOURAGE THE JOINT STABILISERS & CORE MUSCLES TO WORK AS WELL. THIS WAY OF EXERCISING IS DIFFERENT TO THE MATWORK EXERCISES AS YOU HAVE SOMETHING TO PUSH AGAINST, GIVING FEEDBACK TO THE MUSCLES.

The REFORMER supports your body while you exercise lying on a moving platform. The springs can be made lighter or heavier making it more or less difficult

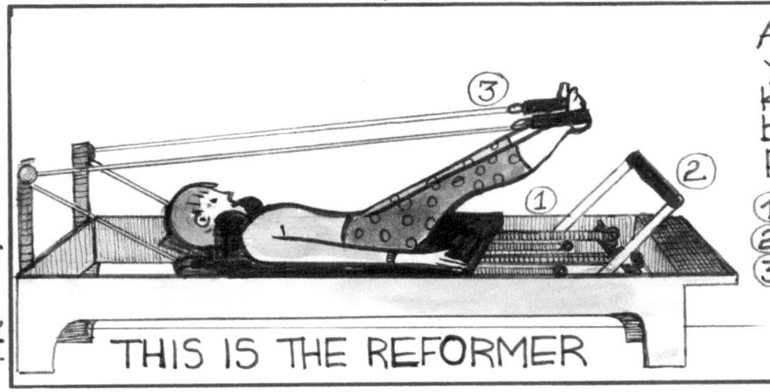
THIS IS THE REFORMER

As well as lying you can also kneel, stand or be in the plank position.

① Springs
② Footbar
③ Leg or Arm straps

Arguably the WUNDACHAIR is the most difficult piece of equipment to master as the body is in an upright position. You have to use your deep abdominal muscles to keep you stable. It can be extremely challenging to do some of the chair exercises needing strength, & flexibility in equal measure.

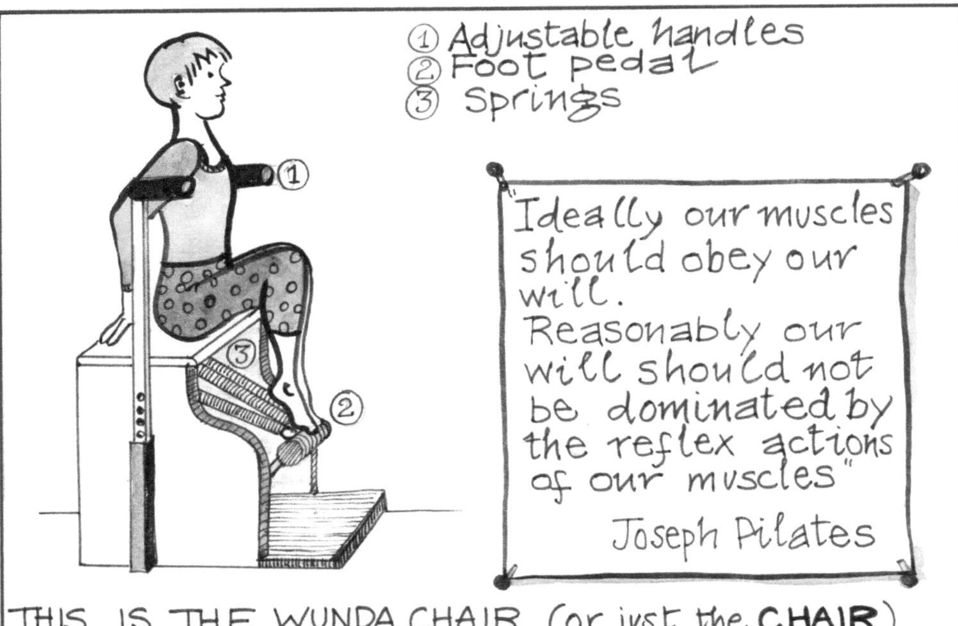

THIS IS THE WUNDA CHAIR (or just the **CHAIR**)

The Essential Characteristics of Pilates (that make it different from any other type of exercise) known as the PRINCIPLES

Breathing

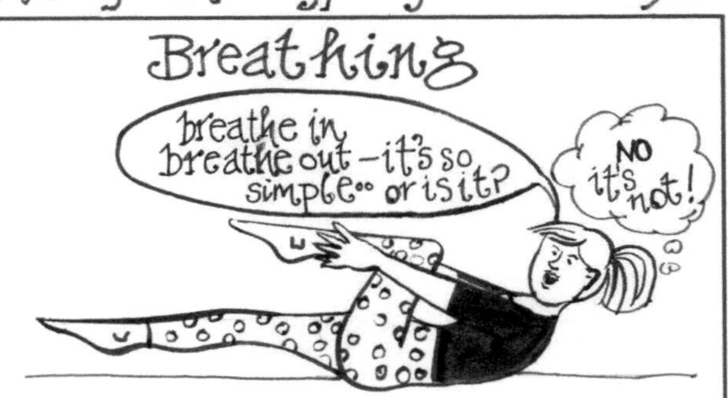

IF YOU ARE BREATHING **CORRECTLY**, TOUGH EXERCISES CAN STILL LEAVE YOU FEELING RELAXED. **BREATHING PROPERLY** OXYGENATES THE BLOOD & INCREASES LUNG CAPACITY.

Flowing Movement

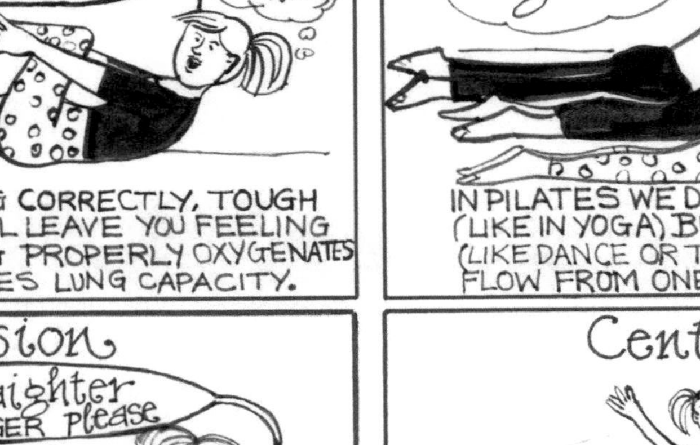

IN PILATES WE DON'T HOLD STATIC POSES (LIKE IN YOGA) BUT MOVE **FREELY** (LIKE DANCE OR TAI CHI). EXERCISES ALSO FLOW FROM ONE TO THE NEXT

Precision

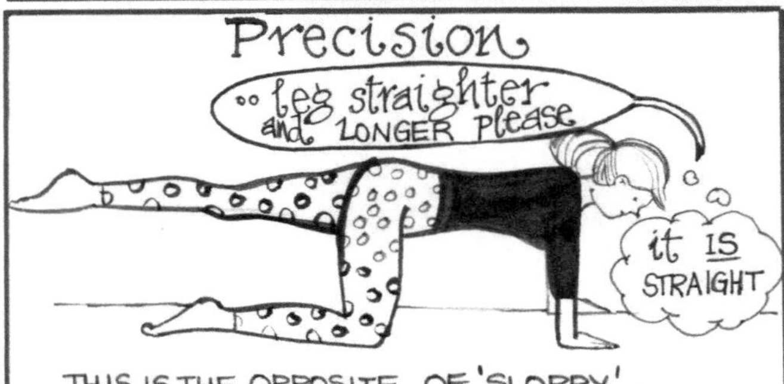

THIS IS THE OPPOSITE OF 'SLOPPY' MOVEMENT! EVERY MOVEMENT IS VERY PRECISE WITH HEAD, BODY & LIMBS IN ALIGNMENT.

Centering

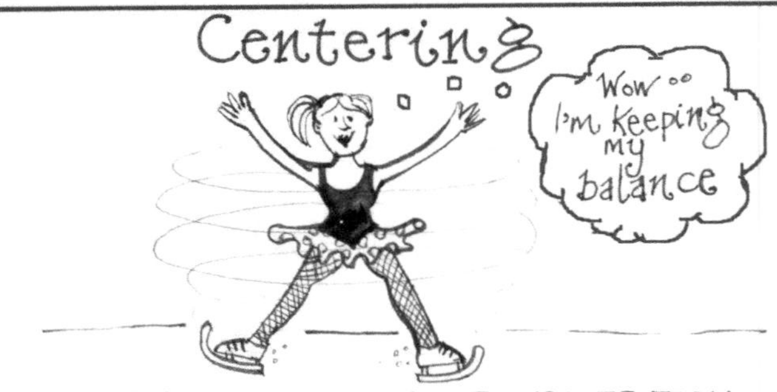

IF YOU ARE CONTROLLING THE MUSCLES FROM THE CENTRE OF YOUR BODY YOU WILL FEEL MORE POWERFUL, HAVE MORE STABILITY & IMPROVE YOUR BALANCE.

Stability

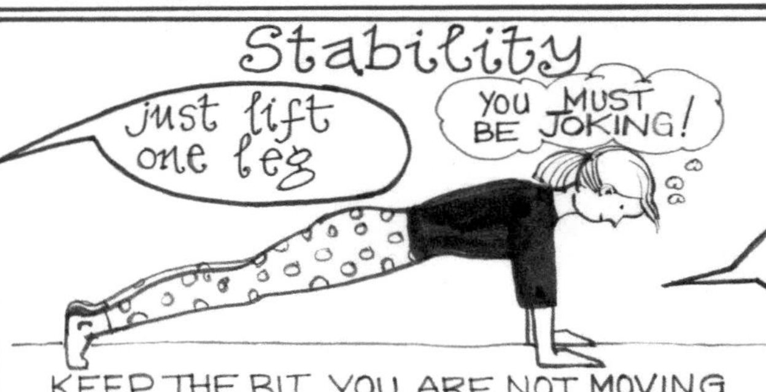

KEEP THE BIT YOU ARE NOT MOVING STABLE & STILL.
LEARNING TO STABILISE YOUR TORSO & SHOULDER GIRDLE HELPS TO PREVENT BACK OR SHOULDER INJURIES.

Control

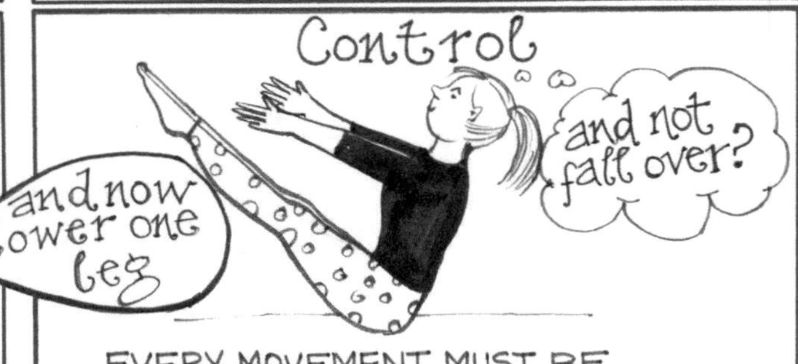

EVERY MOVEMENT MUST BE PERFORMED WITH CONTROL WHETHER YOU ARE LIFTING OR LOWERING YOUR LIMBS OR BENDING & STRAIGHTENING THEM.

Range of Movement

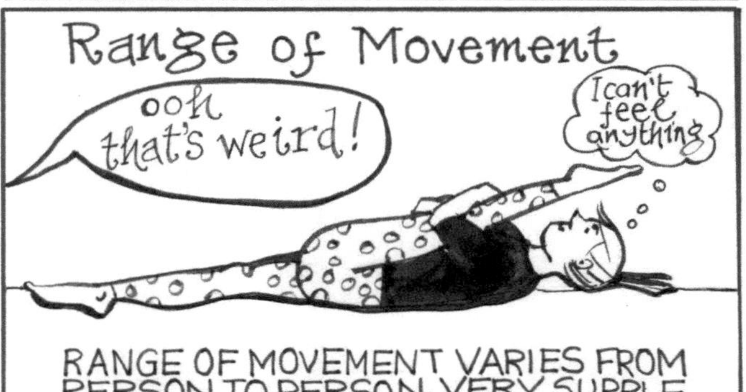

RANGE OF MOVEMENT VARIES FROM PERSON TO PERSON. VERY SUPPLE PEOPLE HAVE TO CONTROL THEIR RANGE OF MOVEMENT.

Opposition

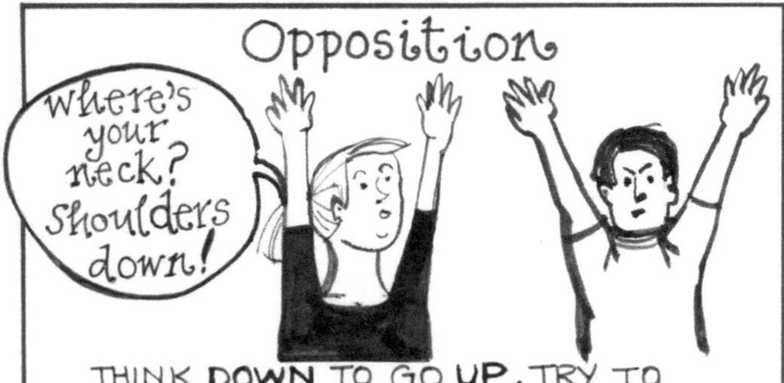

THINK **DOWN** TO GO **UP**. TRY TO KEEP SHOULDERS **DOWN** WHEN THE ARMS LIFT, TUMMY PULLS **UP** AS YOU ROLL **DOWN**. THIS WILL PREVENT INJURY.

Bear in mind that without understanding these principles you are just doing a series of fancy sit-ups & stretches.

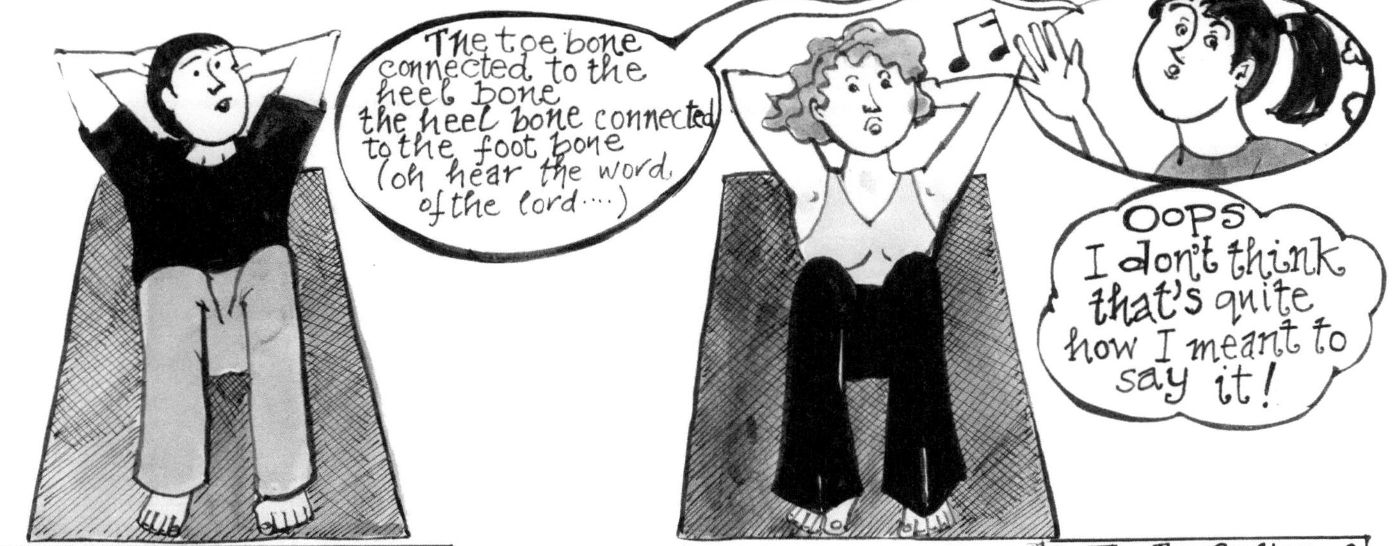

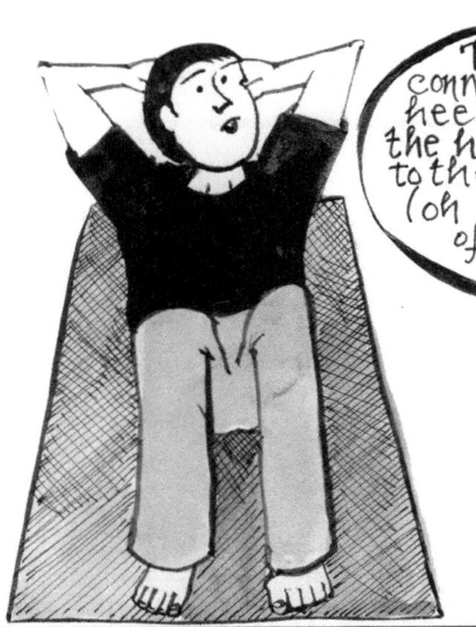

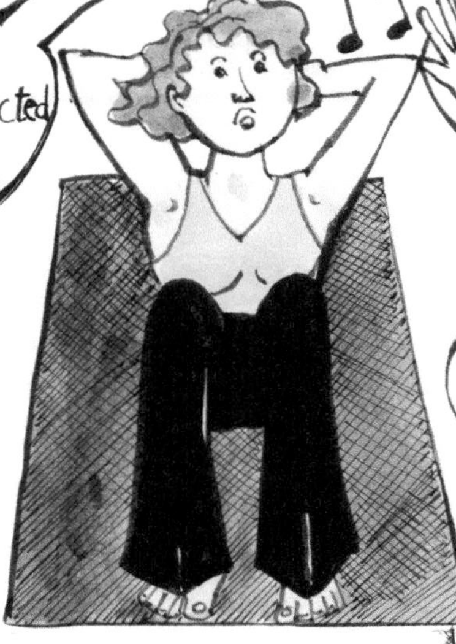

ANATOMY FOR PILATES STUDENTS

...

JUST THE IMPORTANT PARTS

YOU DON'T NEED A DETAILED KNOWLEDGE OF ANATOMY BUT IT HELPS TO KNOW THE NAMES OF THE PARTS OF THE BODY YOUR TEACHER IS TALKING ABOUT & WHERE THEY ARE.

The Two Girdles

The SHOULDER GIRDLE & the PELVIC GIRDLE. They are stacked above each other with a third muscular girdle (the waist) keeping them apart. They turn on the axis of the spine.

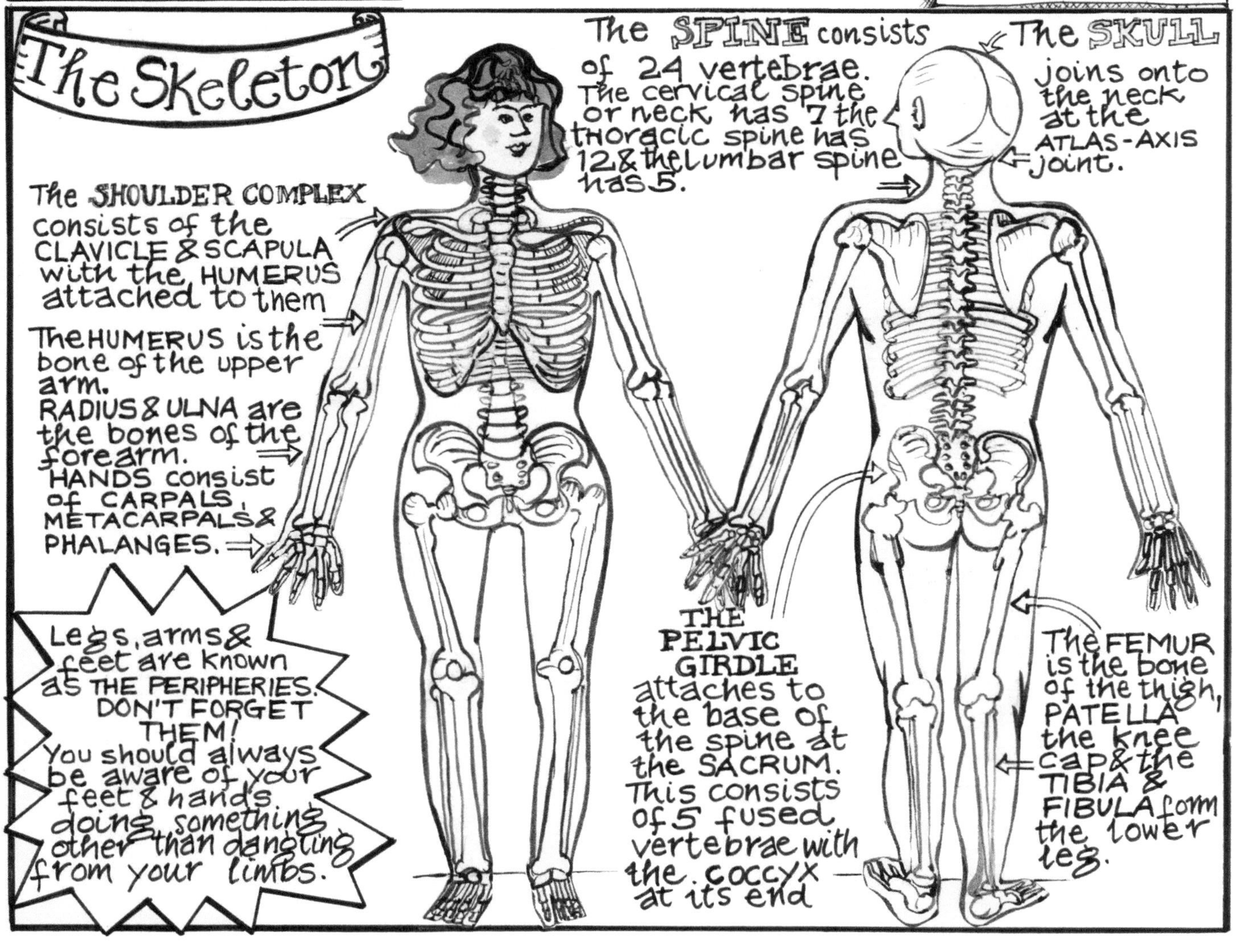

The Skeleton

The SPINE consists of 24 vertebrae. The cervical spine or neck has 7 the thoracic spine has 12 & the lumbar spine has 5.

The SKULL joins onto the neck at the ATLAS-AXIS joint.

The SHOULDER COMPLEX consists of the CLAVICLE & SCAPULA with the HUMERUS attached to them

The HUMERUS is the bone of the upper arm. RADIUS & ULNA are the bones of the forearm. HANDS consist of CARPALS, METACARPALS & PHALANGES.

Legs, arms & feet are known as THE PERIPHERIES. DON'T FORGET THEM! You should always be aware of your feet & hands doing something other than dangling from your limbs.

THE PELVIC GIRDLE attaches to the base of the spine at the SACRUM. This consists of 5 fused vertebrae with the coccyx at its end

The FEMUR is the bone of the thigh, PATELLA the knee cap & the TIBIA & FIBULA form the lower leg.

THE SHOULDER GIRDLE & RIBCAGE

The shoulder girdle consists of a collarbone (**CLAVICLE**) & two shoulder blades (**SCAPULAE**) that fit over the ribcage. The upper arm bone or **HUMERUS** is attached to the shoulder girdle with strong ligaments. Tendons attach the four muscles of the **ROTATOR CUFF** to the **SCAPULA** & **HUMERUS**. These help lift & turn the arm while stabilising the scapula.

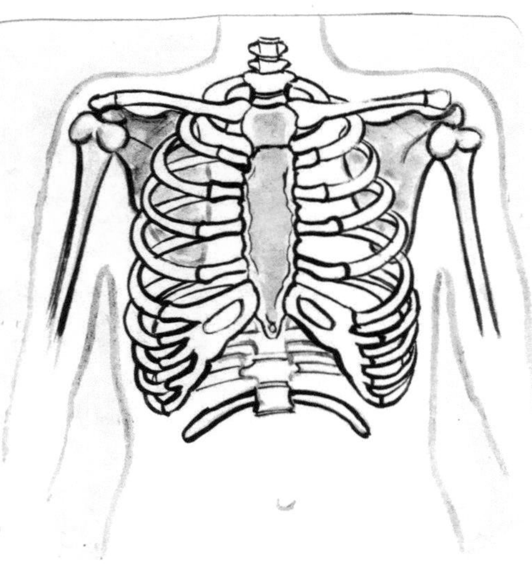

The ribcage protects some of the vital organs such as the **LUNGS & HEART**. It consists of twelve pairs of **RIBS** attached to the **SPINE**. Breathing is the most important means of activating the **INTERCOSTAL MUSCLES** between the ribs. The less we breathe properly the more like a cage it becomes, trapping us in a rigid body.

SCAPULAE (SHOULDER BLADES) ARE USED FOR **STABILISING** THE SHOULDERS WHEN THE ARMS MOVE. THE SHOULDER JOINT IS VERY MOBILE TO ALLOW FOR FREEDOM OF ARM MOVEMENT SO THE ARMS NEED A FIRM ANCHOR. THIS IS DONE BY THE SCAPULAE PULLING TIGHT INTO THE RIBCAGE. HOWEVER THE SCAPULAE ALSO NEED TO HAVE A HEALTHY RANGE OF MOVEMENT

they slide up when you lift your arms

feels smooth & mobile

they slide forwards

they should rest apart

wide & relaxed

shoulder blades glide over the ribcage

Strong & stable shoulderblades should support your bodyweight doing a pressup either against the wall or on the floor without them 'winging'

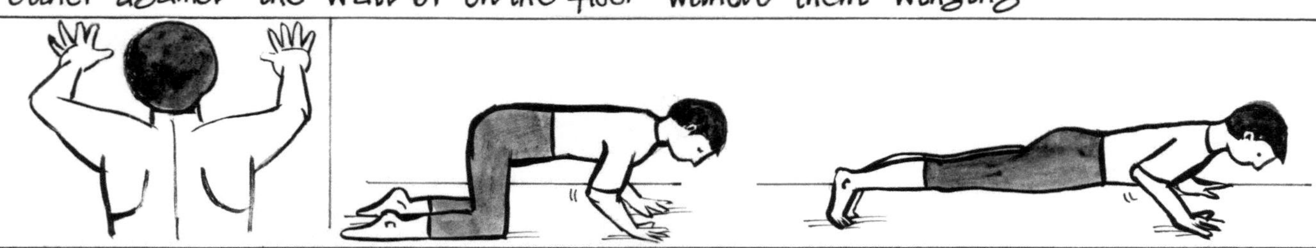

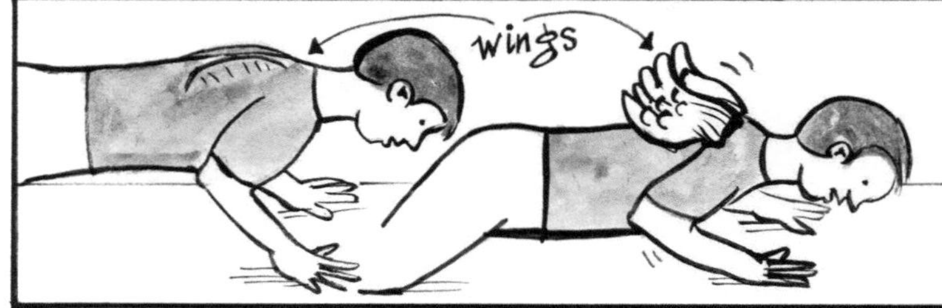

"Winging" is the term for when the shoulder blades pull away from the ribcage & stick out. This may be because the deep shoulder muscles are tight or weak & need to be strengthened with gentle exercises.

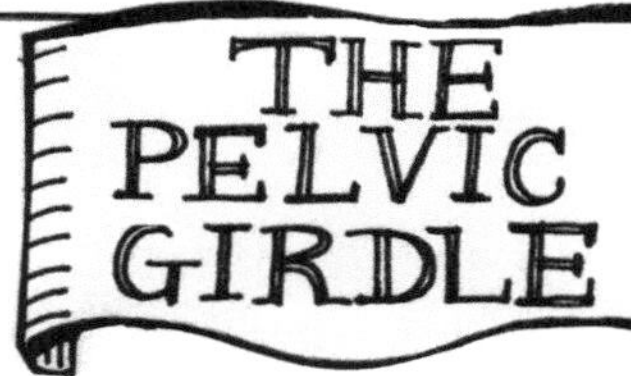

The two biggest bones of the pelvis the ILIUM & the ISCHIUM are joined at the front at the PUBIS (or PUBIC BONE). The base of the spine (SACRUM) is connected to the pelvis at the SACRO ILIAC joint. The PELVIC BASIN is lined with a complex muscular PELVIC FLOOR. One of its functions is to support the viscera & organs. Some of the thigh & back muscles attach to the pelvis.

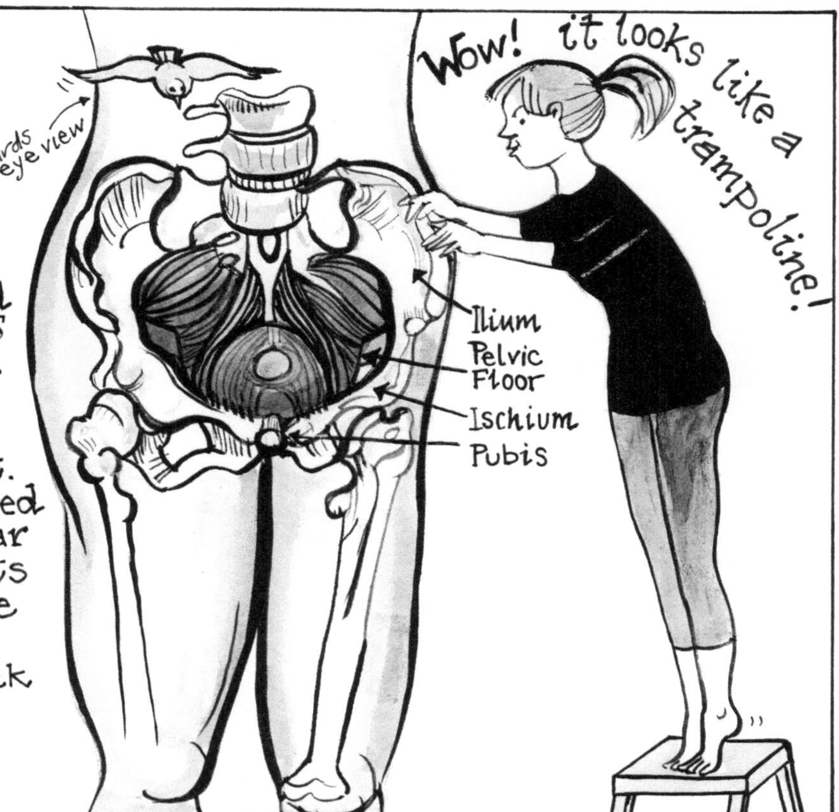

WHERE ARE THE SIT BONES?

When you sit upright on the floor with knees bent you will be resting on two bony lumps, one under each buttock. These useful bony landmarks are the Ischial Tuberosities. Joseph Pilates called them the **SITZ** (SIT) **BONES**.

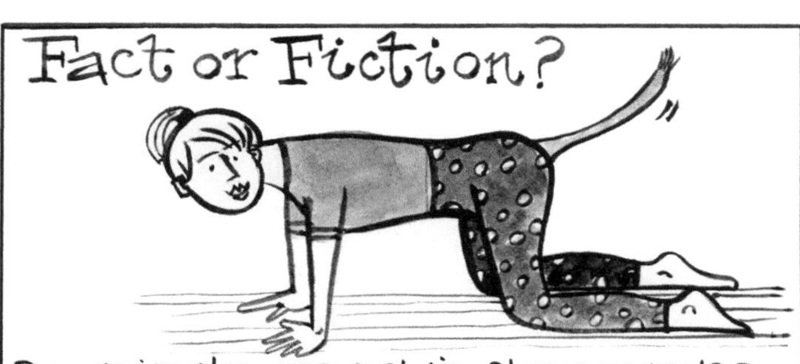

Do animals use pelvic floor muscles to wag their tails? Yes, the Levator Ani muscles are responsible for wagging the tails of **some** quadrupeds

BE AWARE

'A muscle should only be held at about 25% of it's full contraction when not ACTIVELY being recruited.

In other words don't walk around with buttocks clenched, stomach sucked in & pelvic floor lifted at all times

THE PELVIC FLOOR

The primary active function of pelvic floor muscles is to maintain anal & urinary function & in women to facilitate the presentation of the foetus in the birth process

MYTHS ABOUT THE PELVIC FLOOR

The pelvic floor helps you to move

NO!

THE PELVIC FLOOR ASSISTS WITH STABILITY OF THE PELVIS & LOWER SPINE & WORKS TOGETHER WITH THE TRANSVERSUS ABDOMINIS. (SEE BIG 3 ABS)

Does this mean that if you keep your pelvic floor contracted at all times your back will be stronger?

NO!

YOU CAN ONLY HOLD A TRUE PELVIC FLOOR CONTRACTION FOR ABOUT 10 SECONDS AT A TIME. A HEALTHY PELVIC FLOOR SHOULD CONTRACT & BE ABLE TO FULLY RELAX AFTERWARDS.

THE BIG THREE ABDOMINALS

WHY DO WE SPEND SO MUCH TIME FOCUSSING ON ABDOMINAL MUSCLES IN PILATES CLASSES?
IT IS NOT JUST OUT OF VANITY, NOR IS IT IN ORDER TO GET A FLAT TUMMY OR A GOOD 6-PACK. THE MAIN REASON IS THAT THE ABDOMINALS WE NEED TO STRENGTHEN ATTACH TO OUR SPINE & HELP TO SUPPORT US AS WE STAND UPRIGHT & THUS PREVENT POSSIBLE BACK PAIN. THE **GOOD** NEWS IS THAT THESE MUSCLES RESPOND RELATIVELY QUICKLY TO EXERCISE.

Where on earth are they?

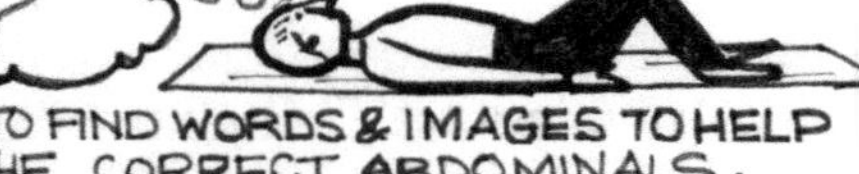

PILATES TEACHERS SPEND AN INORDINATE AMOUNT OF TIME TRYING TO FIND WORDS & IMAGES TO HELP STUDENTS "RECRUIT" (FIND & USE) THE CORRECT ABDOMINALS. (SUCK IN YOUR GUT!) HOWEVER THE RESULTS CAN BE A LITTLE CONFUSING.
OUR AIM IS TO ACTIVATE A GROUP OF ELUSIVE MUSCLES & CALM THE MORE DOMINANT ONES.

The Simpletons Guide to Locating the ABDOMINAL MUSCLES

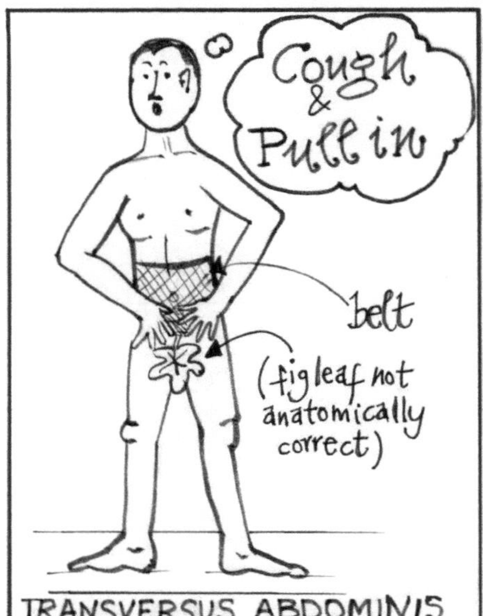

TRANSVERSUS ABDOMINIS
Imagine a wide elastic belt

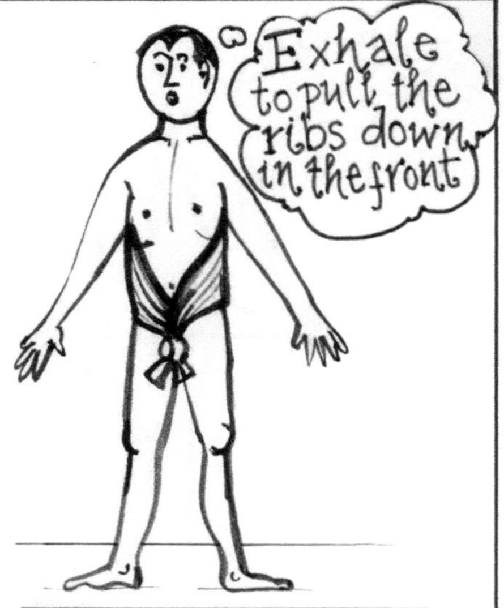

INTERNAL & EXTERNAL OBLIQUES
Imagine a shawl wrapped around the back knotted at the pubic bone

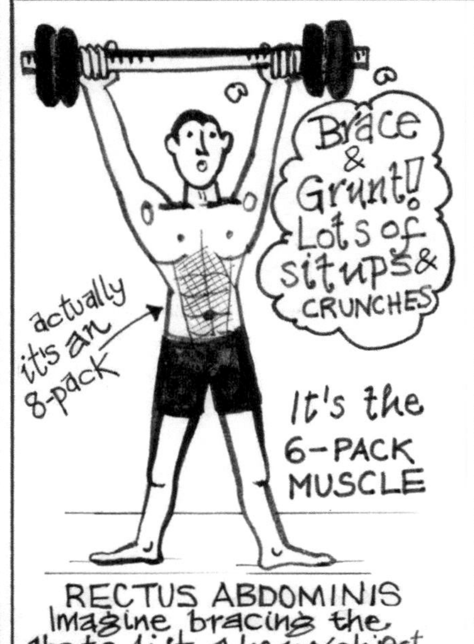

RECTUS ABDOMINIS
Imagine bracing the abs to lift a heavy object

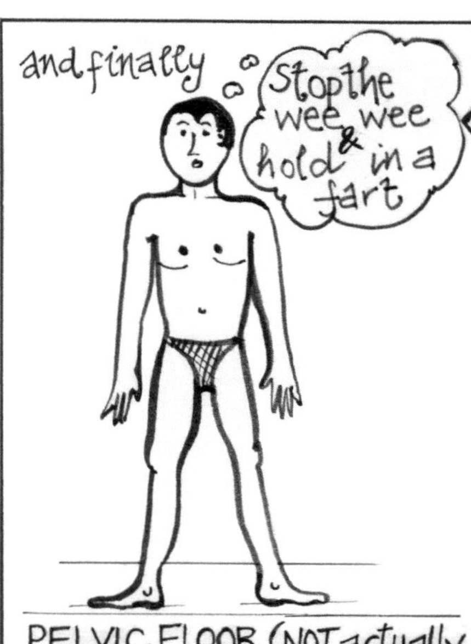

PELVIC FLOOR (NOT actually an Ab)
Imagine a thong a size too small

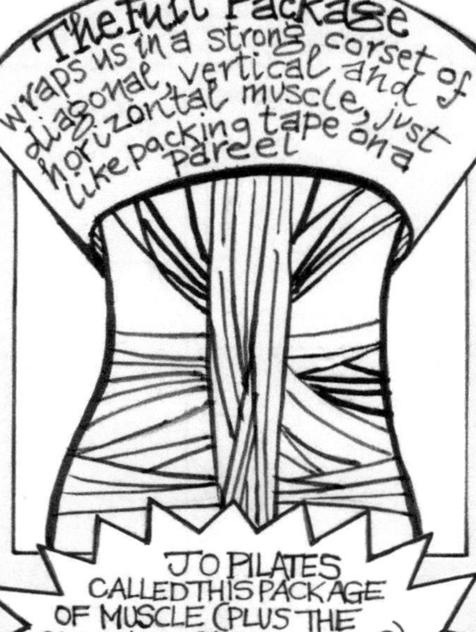

J.O PILATES CALLED THIS PACKAGE OF MUSCLE (PLUS THE GLUTEALS & BACK MUSCLES) THE POWER HOUSE (or probably Das Power Haus as he was German)

TO HAVE GOOD POSTURE ONE NEEDS STRONG TUMMY MUSCLES. TRY SITTING UPRIGHT ON A STOOL, THE HEAD BALANCED ABOVE THE HIPS & LOOK AHEAD

FEEL HOW THE TUMMY CONTRACTS TO HOLD THE SPINE FROM THE FRONT WHILE THE BACK MUSCLES SUPPORT IT FROM BEHIND. THIS IS LIKE WEARING A SUPPORTIVE GIRDLE.

ASK CORA TO HELP YOU ANSWER YOUR PILATES QUESTIONS

Dear Cora, I read that you can strengthen your abs by doing crunches every day but I am getting nowhere. Am I doing something wrong?

What have you been reading? OVERTRAINING WEEKLY? Old school ab exercises such as THE CRUNCH neglect the muscles responsible for holding your posture upright & those that stabilise your joints. Doing crunches every day will overwork Rectus Abdominis. It needs time to recover!

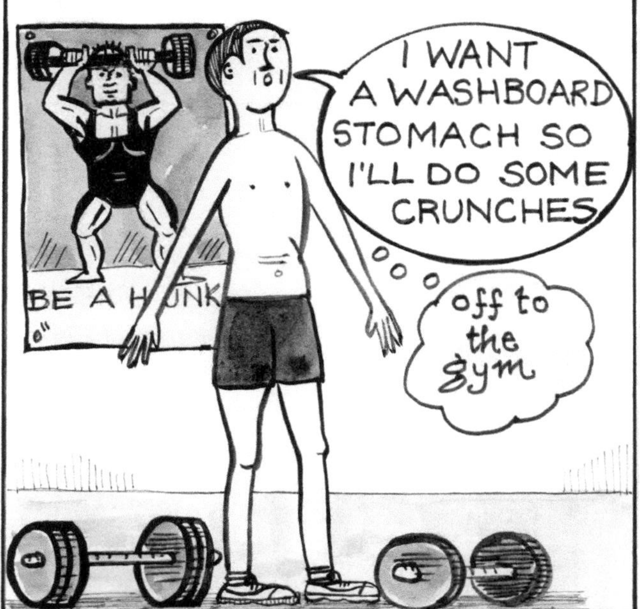

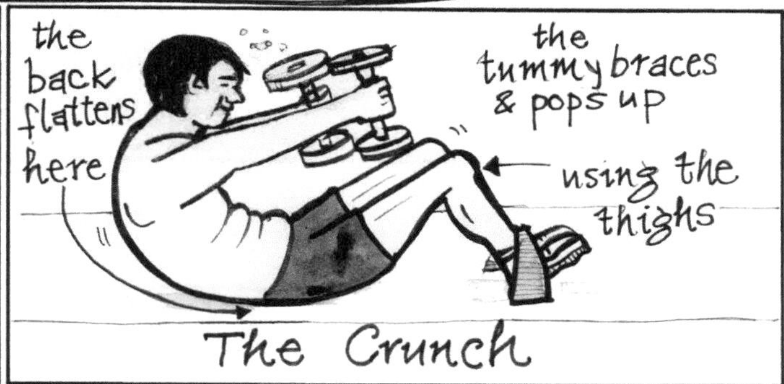

The Crunch

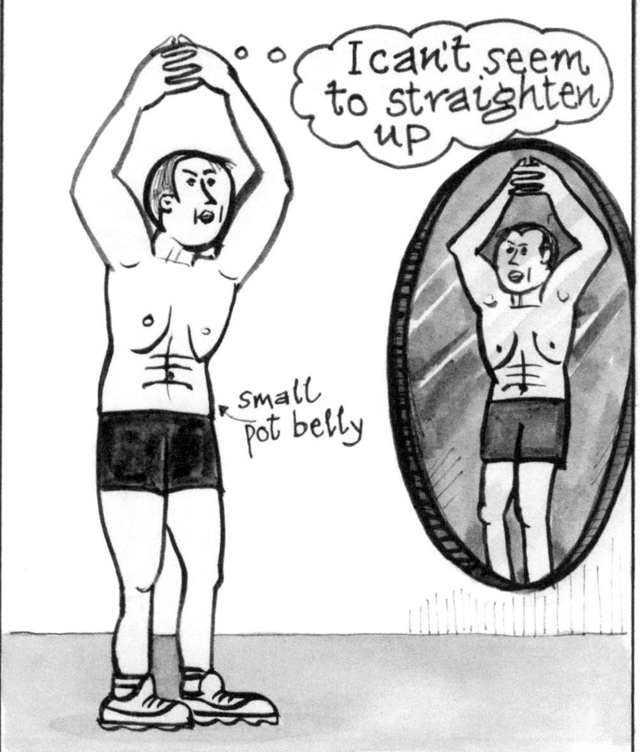

Doing repeated crunches will strengthen RECTUS ABDOMINIS the SIX PACK MUSCLE but tightening this muscle in isolation can pull you forward & you may appear stooped. If you also strengthen the deep abdominal muscles these will create a girdle of support for the spine. The AB-CURL may look similar but is a totally different exercise. The pace is slower & the movement feels more intense. It eliminates any momentum & activates deep stabilising abdominals. This may LOOK easy, but don't be fooled! The AB-CURL will challenge you in a different way.

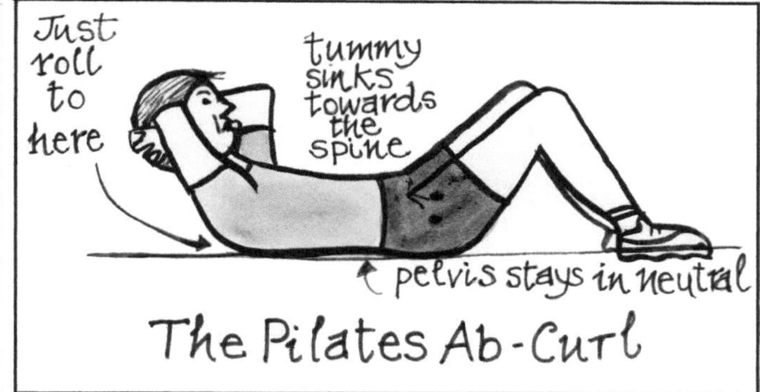

The Pilates Ab-Curl

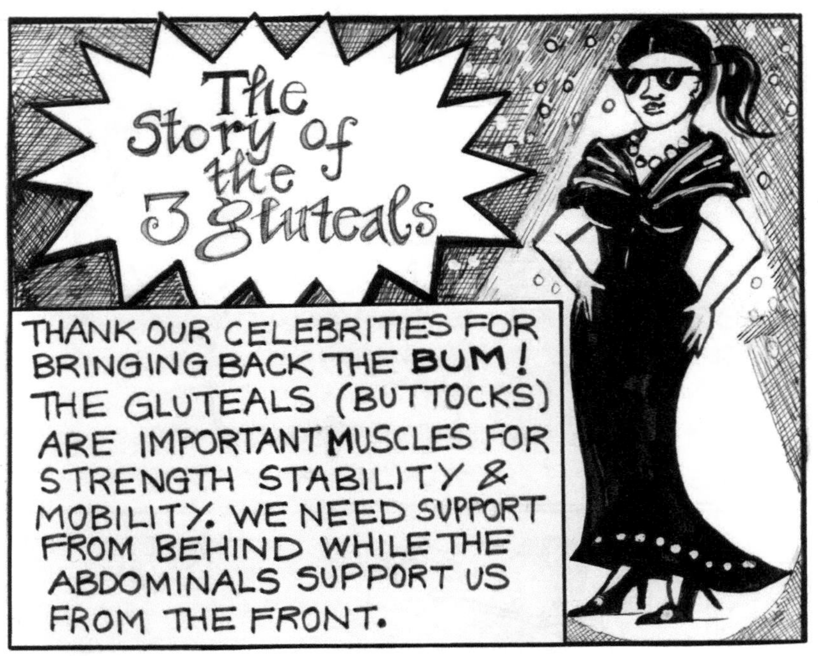

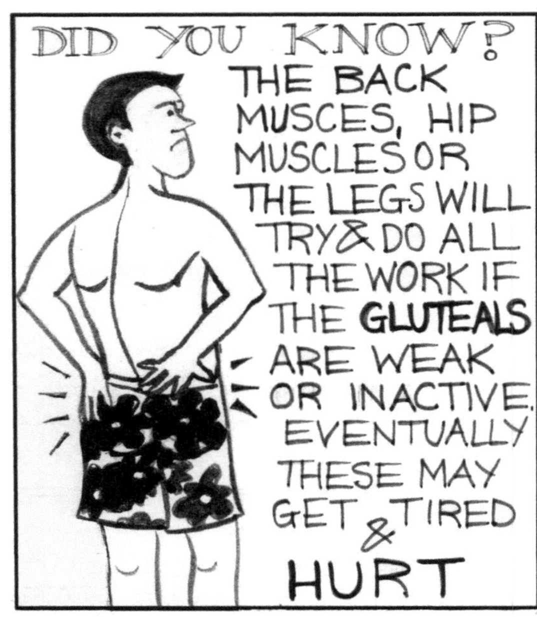

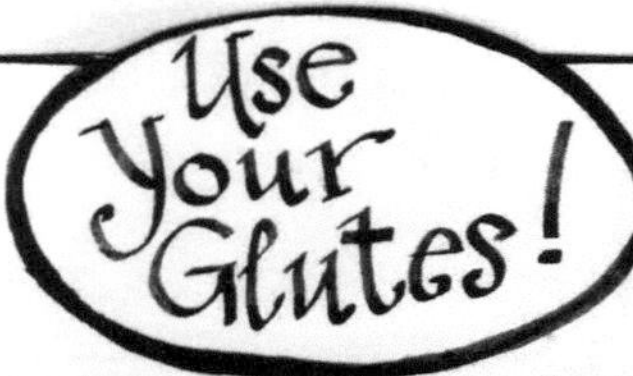

IS A COMMAND THAT MAY MAKE YOU CLENCH YOUR BUTTOCKS! TRY WALKING LIKE THAT & YOU'LL BE A LITTLE STIFF-LEGGED. A PILATES TEACHER IS TUNED TO SPOT IF YOU ARE USING YOUR GLUTEALS DURING EXERCISES & TRAINED TO HELP YOU SWITCH ON THE CORRECT ONES AS WELL AS TO SWITCH THEM OFF AGAIN.

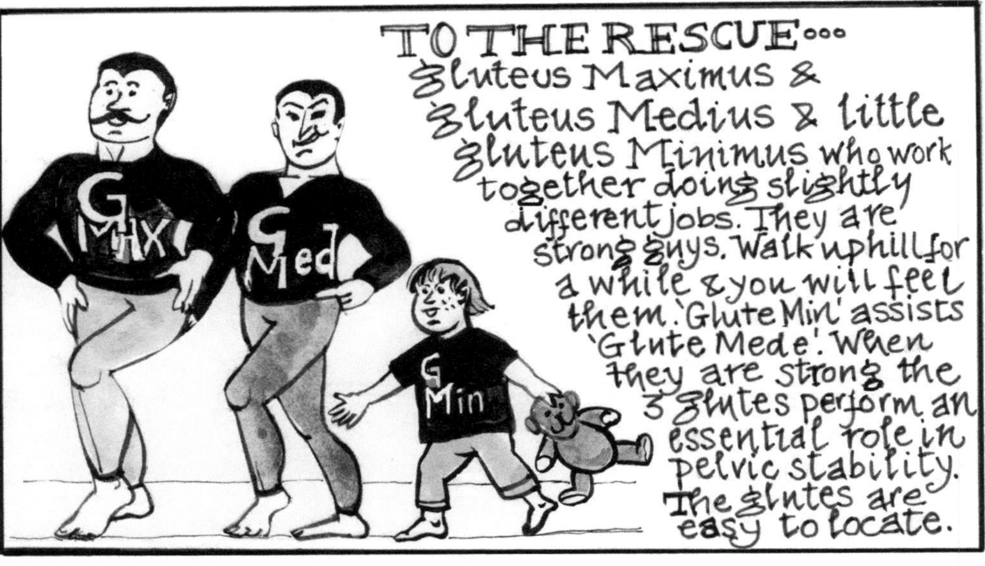

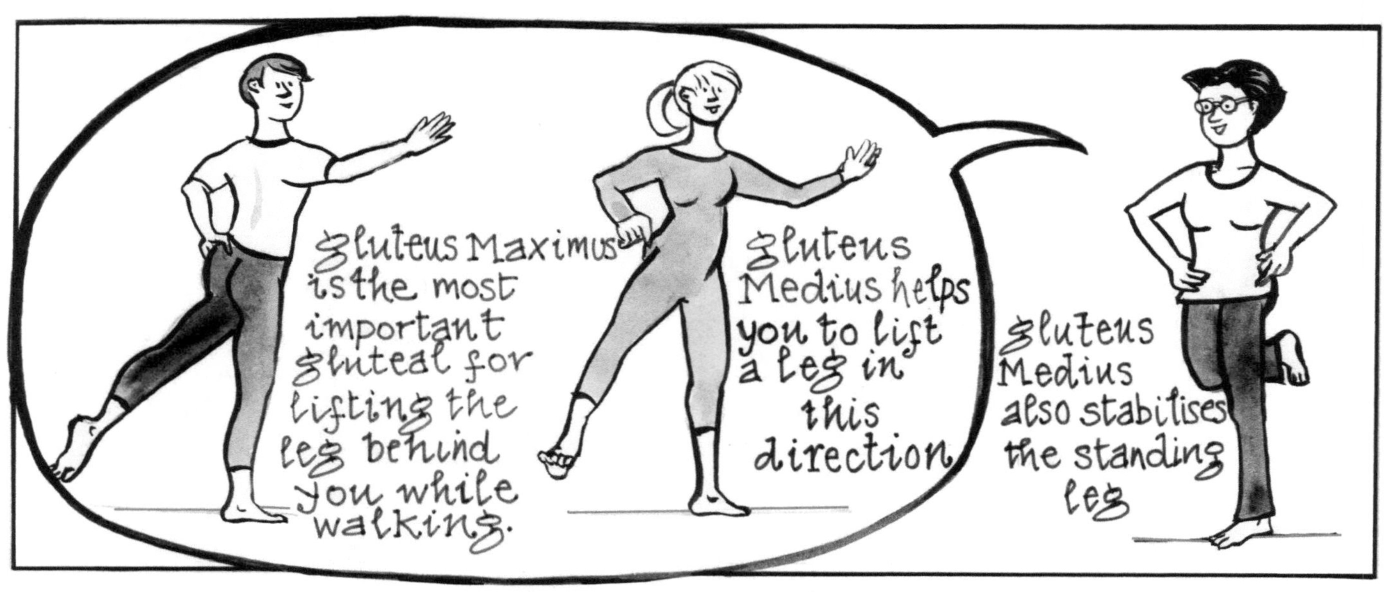

HOW TO FIND GLUTEUS MAXIMUS

Exercises to strengthen the gluteals don't have to be dramatic to be effective. This is a simple way to find glute Max & work it hard. Just make sure that you don't bend your knees or lift your leg more than two inches off the floor.

① Lie with the tips of the toes just touching a wall. Engage your abs, anchoring the pelvis. Reach for the wall & try to lift the kneecap & thigh with a straight leg

② Engage abs, flex feet & squeeze heels together with straight legs. Open & close legs to squeeze six times.

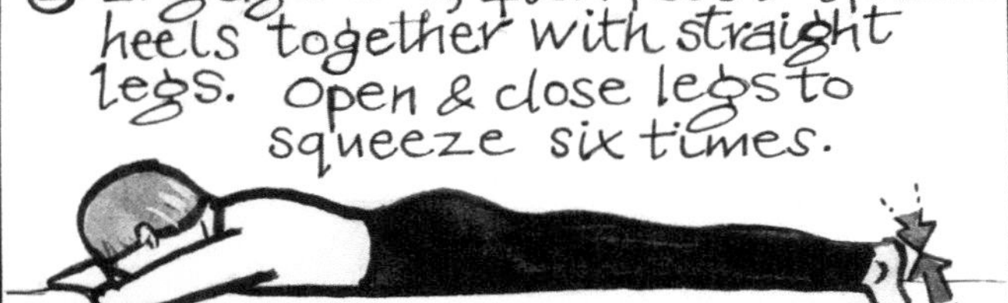

③ Lift abdominals. (as in no1) Reach with one leg & lift straight leg approximately 2 inches then lower it

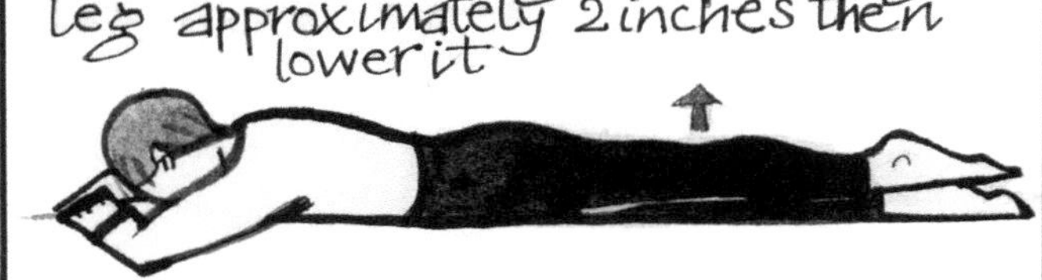

④ alternate legs in a slow swimming action, legs VERY straight.

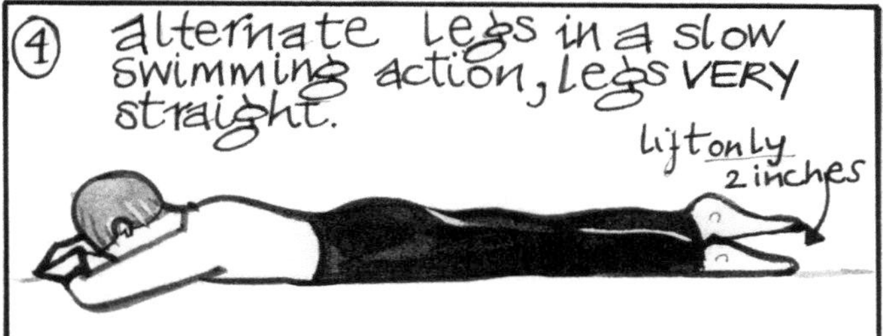

The Hips & gluteals need regular stretching. The first three exercises are great but don't do them if you have had a hip replacement. They also stretch the muscles around your knees but they will gradually become used to it. Daily stretches will make your hips more flexible.

Lie on your back & cross your legs above the knees as if sitting on a bar stool. Hug the back of your knees & as you exhale, squeeze your legs tightly in towards you. Hold & slowly release on 3 counts. Repeat with the other leg on top.

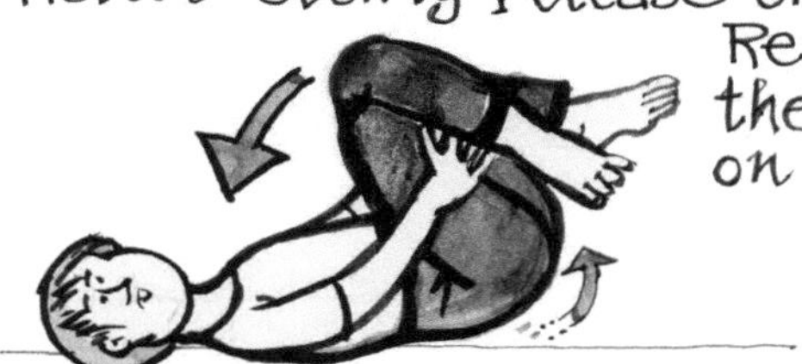

①

Cross your legs with the ankle above the knee, as if in the yoga half lotus position. Slide your arms between your legs & hug them towards you. Try to keep your knees level. Hold & slowly release. Repeat with the other leg on top.

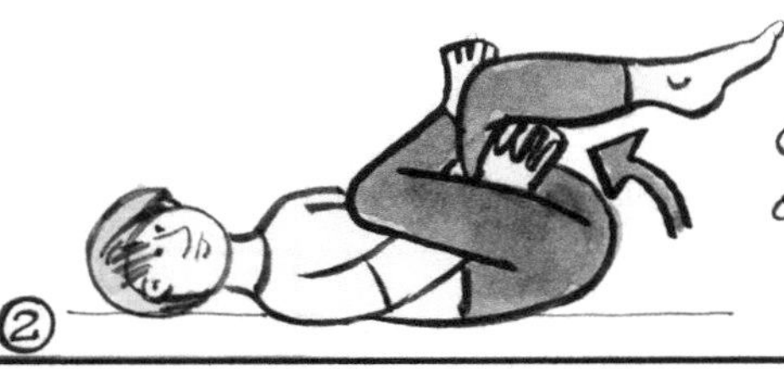

②

③ With a bent leg place the side of your ankle & knee on the arm of a sofa. Lean forward slowly over your bent leg taking the weight on your arms. Hold this position. Repeat with the other leg.

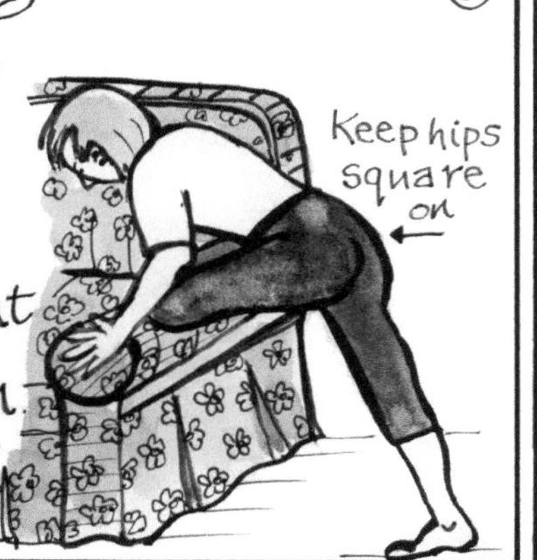

If you have had a hip replacement or just have muscle tightness, place a tennis ball on the wall behind your buttock. Lean your weight into it and roll it up & down about 10 times on the tight area.

Repeat regularly

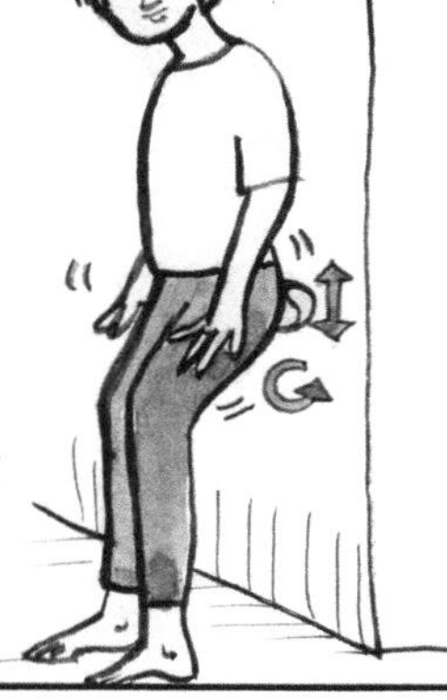

THE UNIVERSAL CRY IN A PILATES CLASS IS...

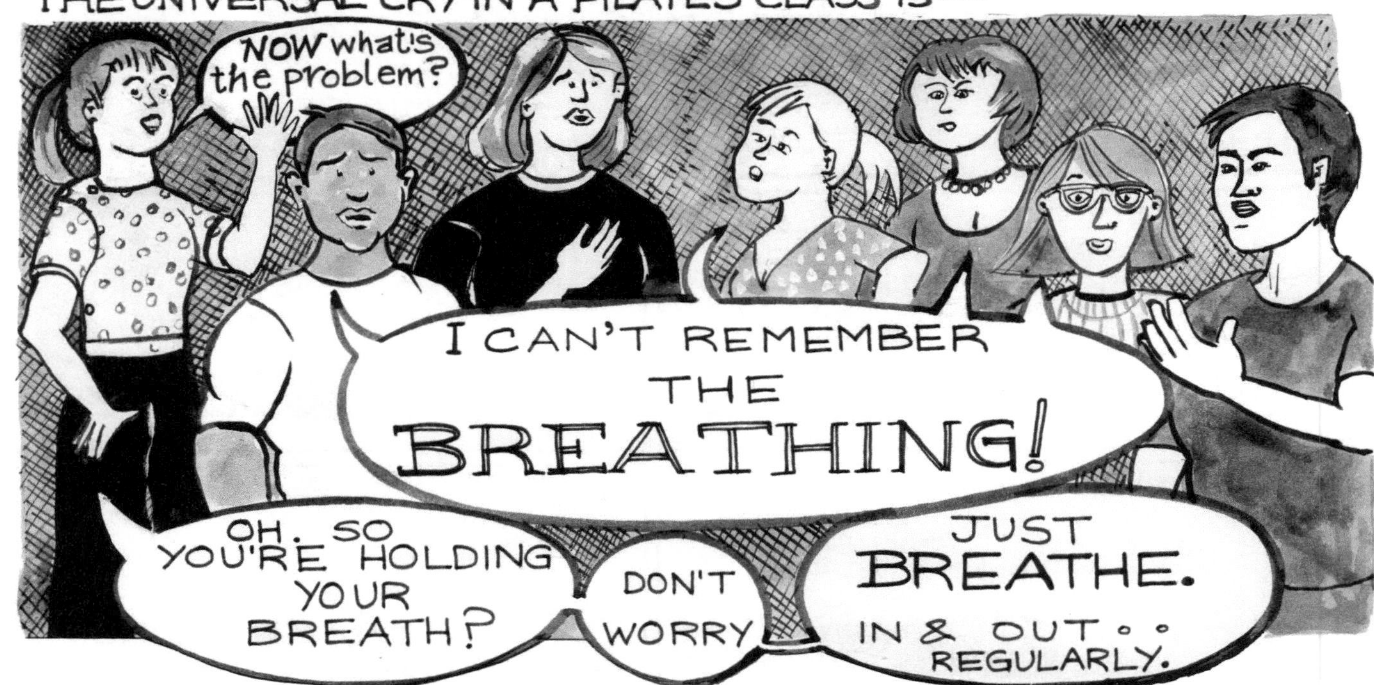

BREATHING is the magic & vital ingredient in Pilates. A little like baking powder in a cake mix, the shape & taste of the end product is similar but the quality of LIGHTNESS is missing. Breathing correctly while doing the exercises will make them & your body come alive. Aches can vanish & seemingly impossible movements become possible. At the end of class you have more energy than when you began. Not only does breathing oxygenate the blood but the action of the ribcage expanding & contracting helps to increase flexibility.

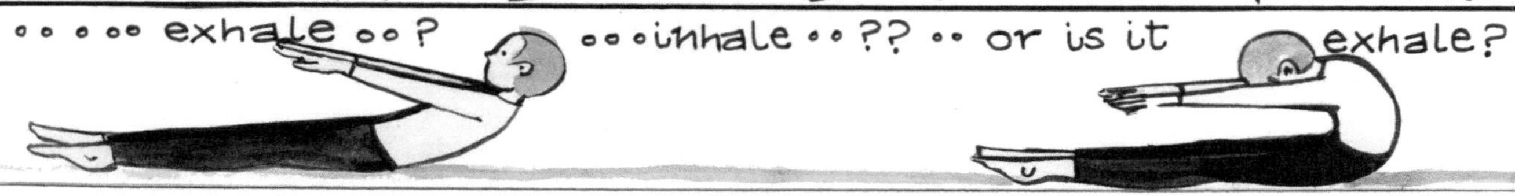

In Pilates exercises there is a general rule that movements that require more effort are done on the exhale. It is more likely that you will 'pop' your abdominals whilst inhaling, thus losing stability & strength. However rules are made to be broken & teachers will often challenge you by changing the breathing in the exercises.

LATERAL BREATHING

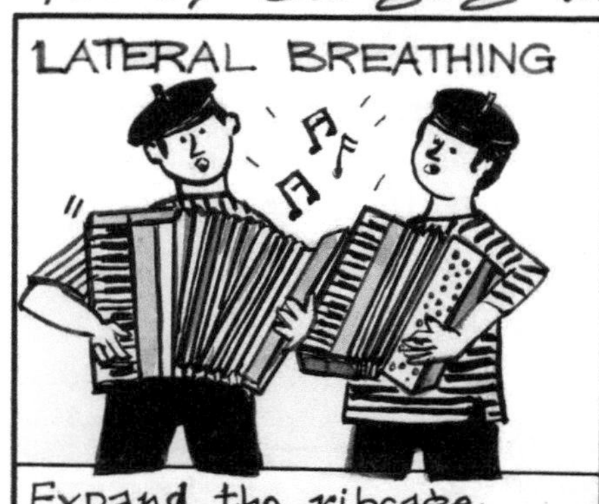

Expand the ribcage widthways as you inhale. Squeeze all the air out as you exhale (like an accordion)

PERCUSSIVE BREATHING

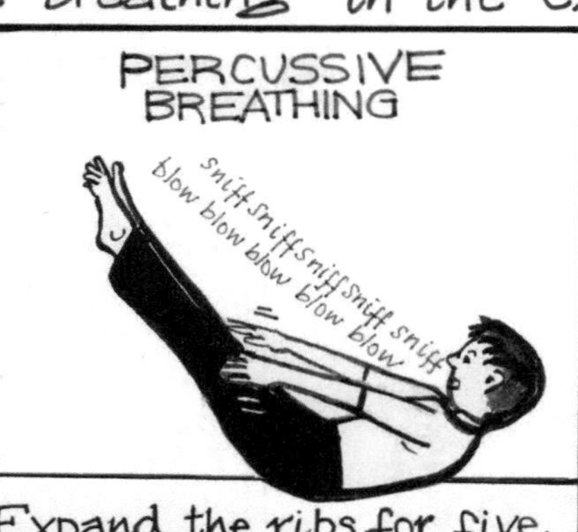

Expand the ribs for five sharp inbreaths & exhale for five sharp outbreaths. You use this in the HUNDREDS

HIDE & SEEK BREATHING

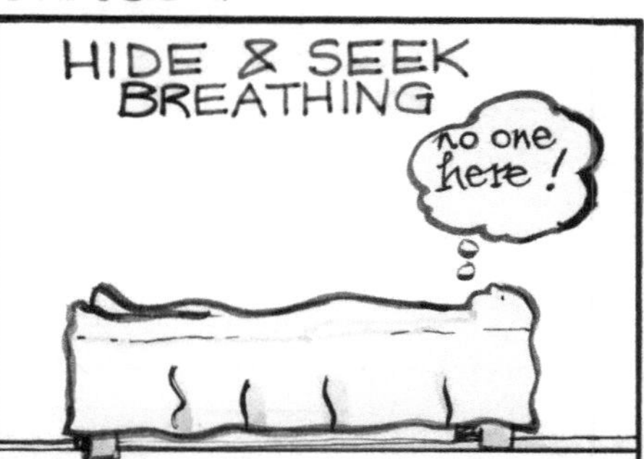

Imagine you're hiding under a sheet & can't breathe too deeply in case you are discovered. Use this if you don't want to pop the abs.

Above
all
Learn how
to
BREATHE
properly

Joseph Pilates

Working in harmony with the muscular system is the NERVOUS SYSTEM that sends impulses to the muscles from both the conscious & the unconscious mind. The MIND & BODY are like an old fashioned telephone exchange where the BRAIN sends messages down the wires (NERVES) to the BODY. It may take time to establish, but once the connections are made & messages are passing along the wires our bodies rarely completely forget learned actions. We can then continue to activate more subtle wiring in order to refine our movements & become better at what we do.

THE MORE YOU USE THEM THE STRONGER THE PATHWAYS BECOME UNTIL THEY ARE MORE LIKE HIGHWAYS THAN PATHS. EXAMPLES ARE USING YOUR HANDS TO PLAY THE PIANO OR EVEN THE ABILITY TO LIFT THE INDIVIDUAL TOES OF YOUR FEET.

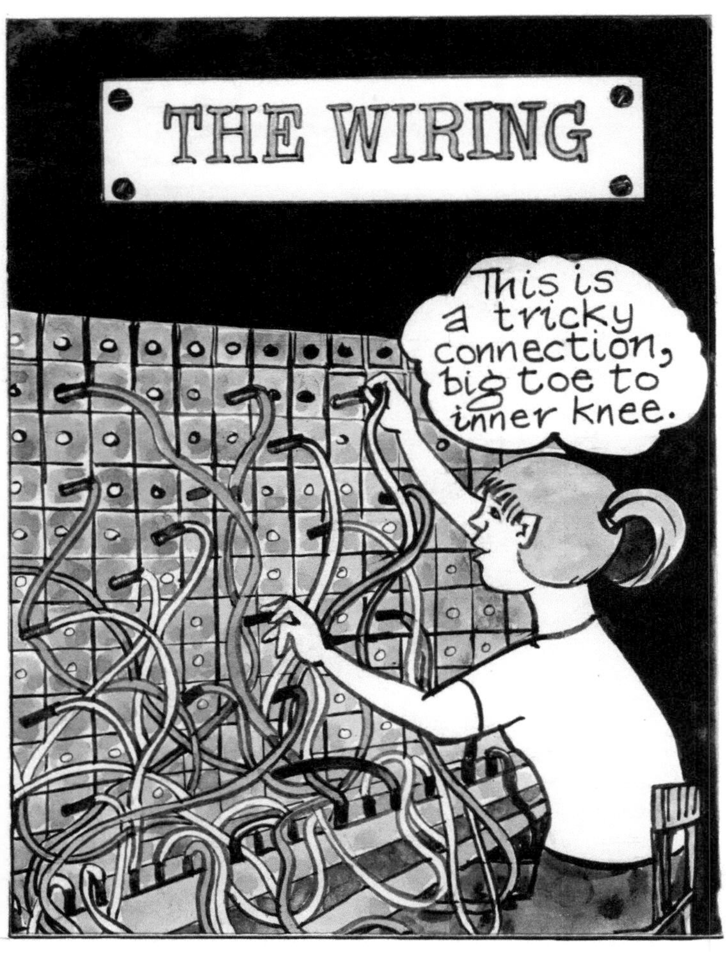

As beginners our brains are working overtime & we often feel we are 'not doing it right'. Then there are the lightbulb moments when it all comes together & the exercises seem effortless.

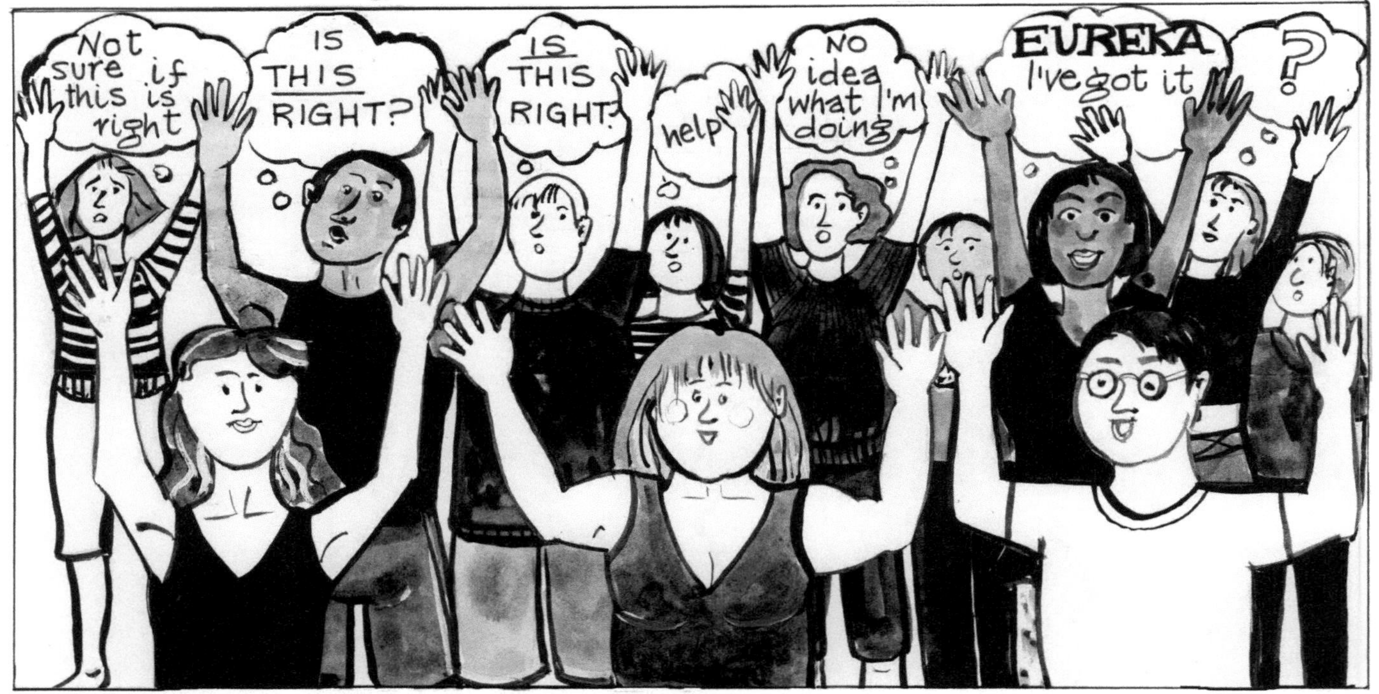

By the time we have been doing Pilates for some time the majority of the movements will have become AUTOMATIC & relegated to the parts of the brain dealing with routine tasks.

THE AUTONOMIC NERVOUS SYSTEM

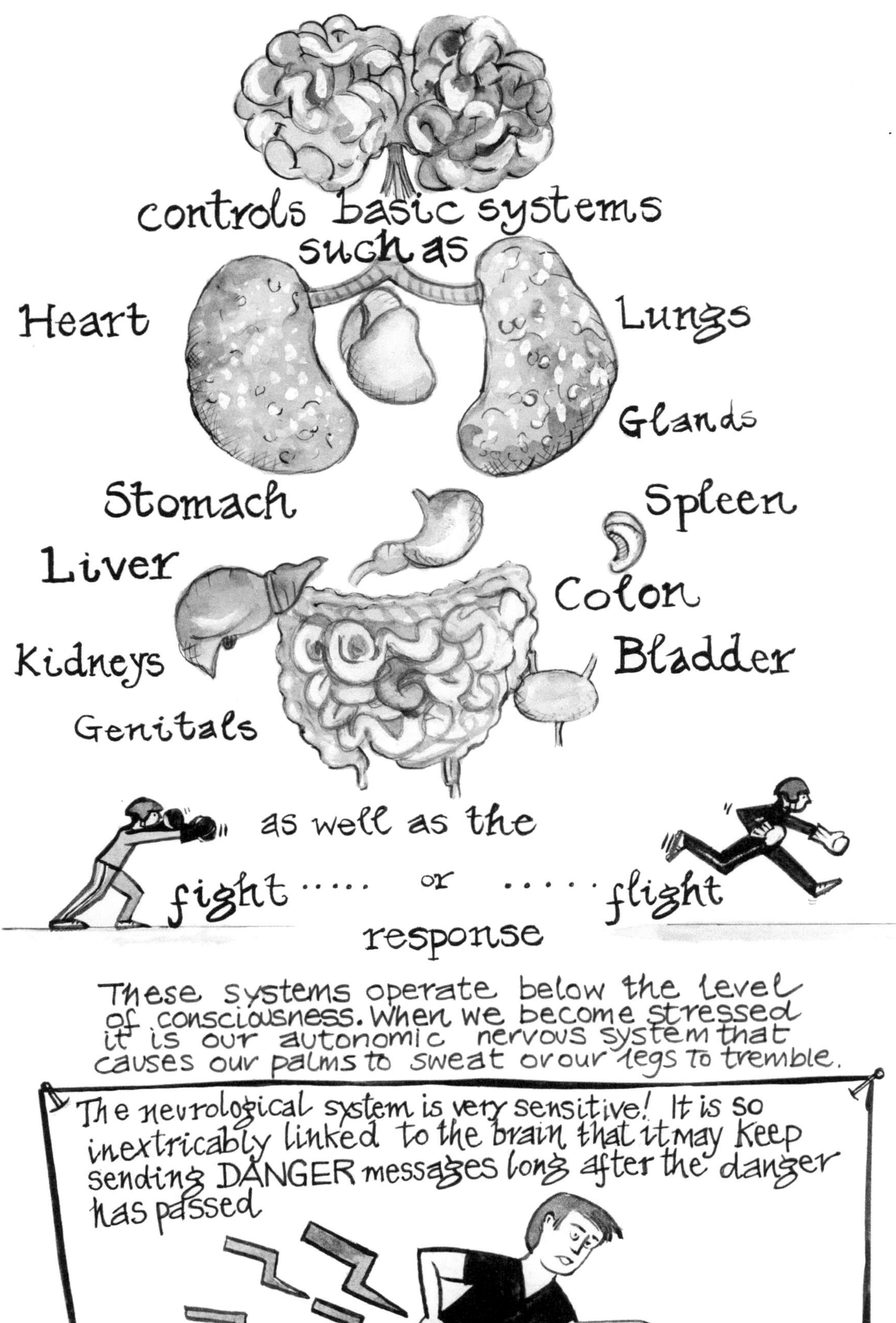

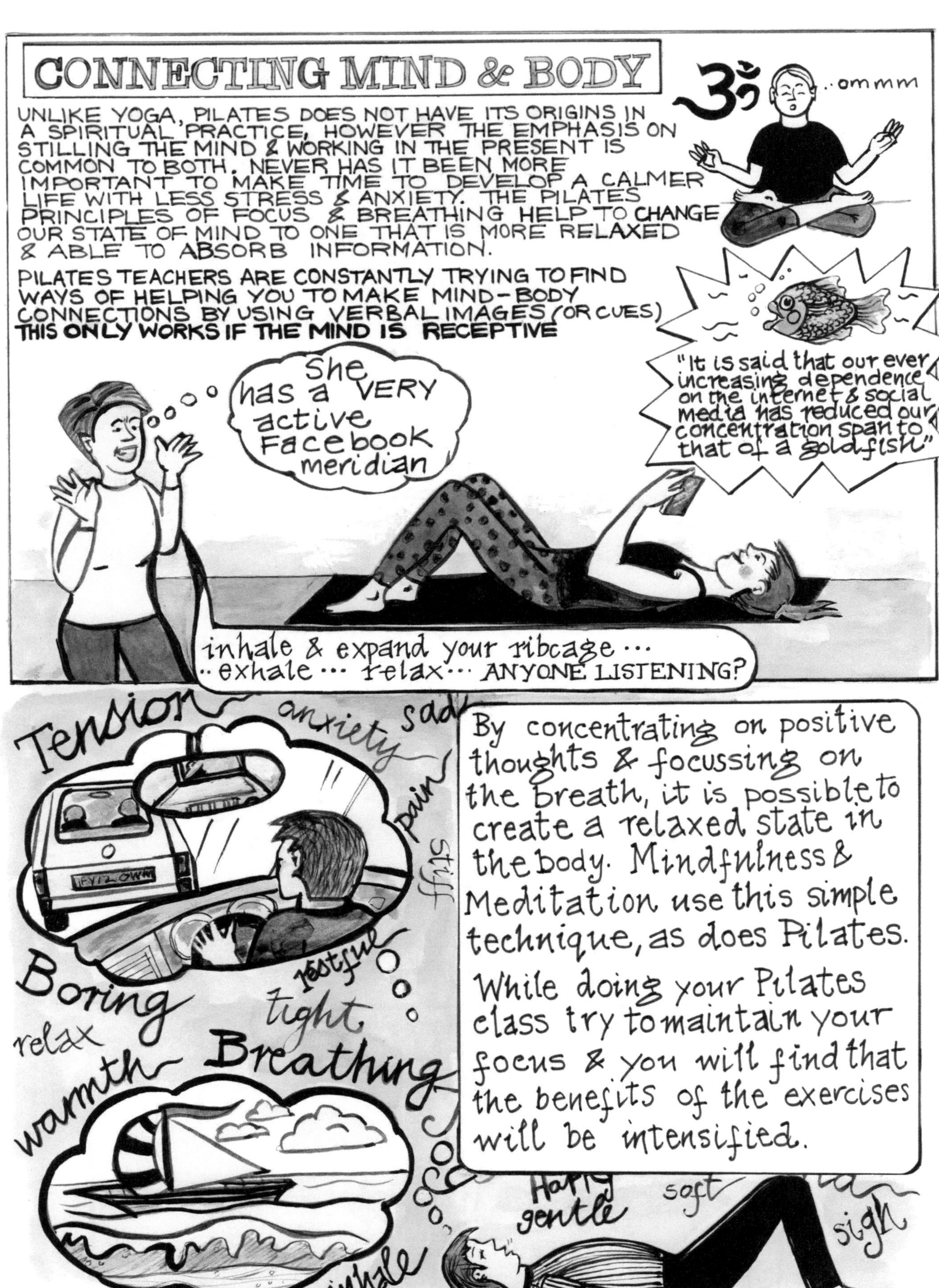

CONNECTING MIND & BODY
UNLIKE YOGA, PILATES DOES NOT HAVE ITS ORIGINS IN A SPIRITUAL PRACTICE, HOWEVER THE EMPHASIS ON STILLING THE MIND & WORKING IN THE PRESENT IS COMMON TO BOTH. NEVER HAS IT BEEN MORE IMPORTANT TO MAKE TIME TO DEVELOP A CALMER LIFE WITH LESS STRESS & ANXIETY. THE PILATES PRINCIPLES OF FOCUS & BREATHING HELP TO CHANGE OUR STATE OF MIND TO ONE THAT IS MORE RELAXED & ABLE TO ABSORB INFORMATION.
PILATES TEACHERS ARE CONSTANTLY TRYING TO FIND WAYS OF HELPING YOU TO MAKE MIND-BODY CONNECTIONS BY USING VERBAL IMAGES (OR CUES)
THIS ONLY WORKS IF THE MIND IS RECEPTIVE
..ommm
"It is said that our ever increasing dependence on the internet & social media has reduced our concentration span to that of a goldfish"
She has a VERY active Facebook meridian
inhale & expand your ribcage... ..exhale... relax... ANYONE LISTENING?
Tension
anxiety
sad
pain
stiff
restful
Boring
tight
relax
warmth
Breathing
By concentrating on positive thoughts & focussing on the breath, it is possible to create a relaxed state in the body. Mindfulness & Meditation use this simple technique, as does Pilates.
While doing your Pilates class try to maintain your focus & you will find that the benefits of the exercises will be intensified.
Happy
gentle
soft
sigh
inhale

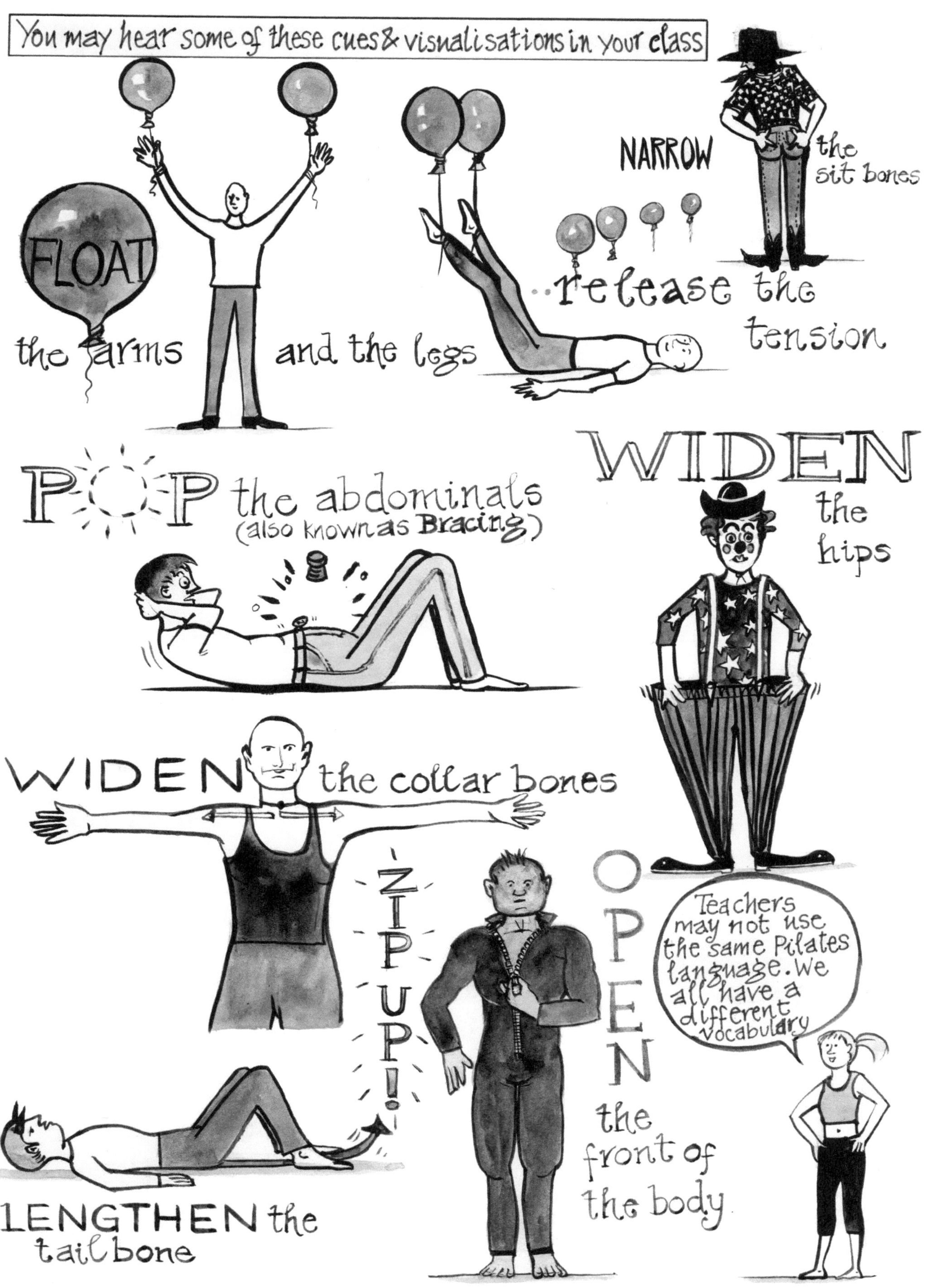
You may hear some of these cues & visualisations in your class
FLOAT
the arms
and the legs
release the tension
NARROW the sit bones
POP the abdominals
(also known as Bracing)
WIDEN the hips
WIDEN the collar bones
ZIP UP!
OPEN the front of the body
Teachers may not use the same Pilates language. We all have a different vocabulary
LENGTHEN the tailbone

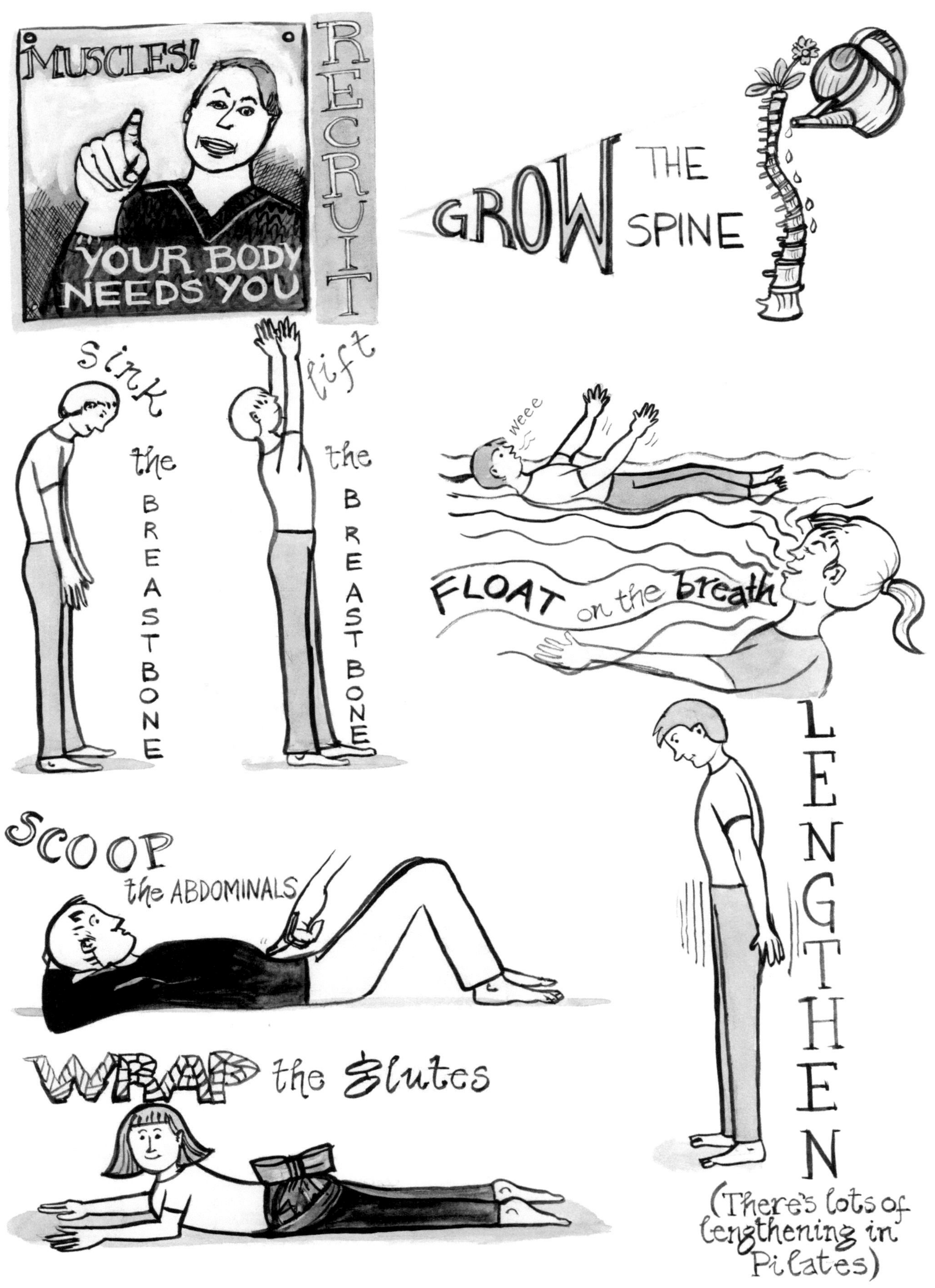
MUSCLES!
YOUR BODY NEEDS YOU
RECRUIT
GROW THE SPINE
sink the BREASTBONE
lift the BREASTBONE
weee
FLOAT on the breath
LENGTHEN
(There's lots of lengthening in Pilates)
SCOOP the ABDOMINALS
WRAP the glutes

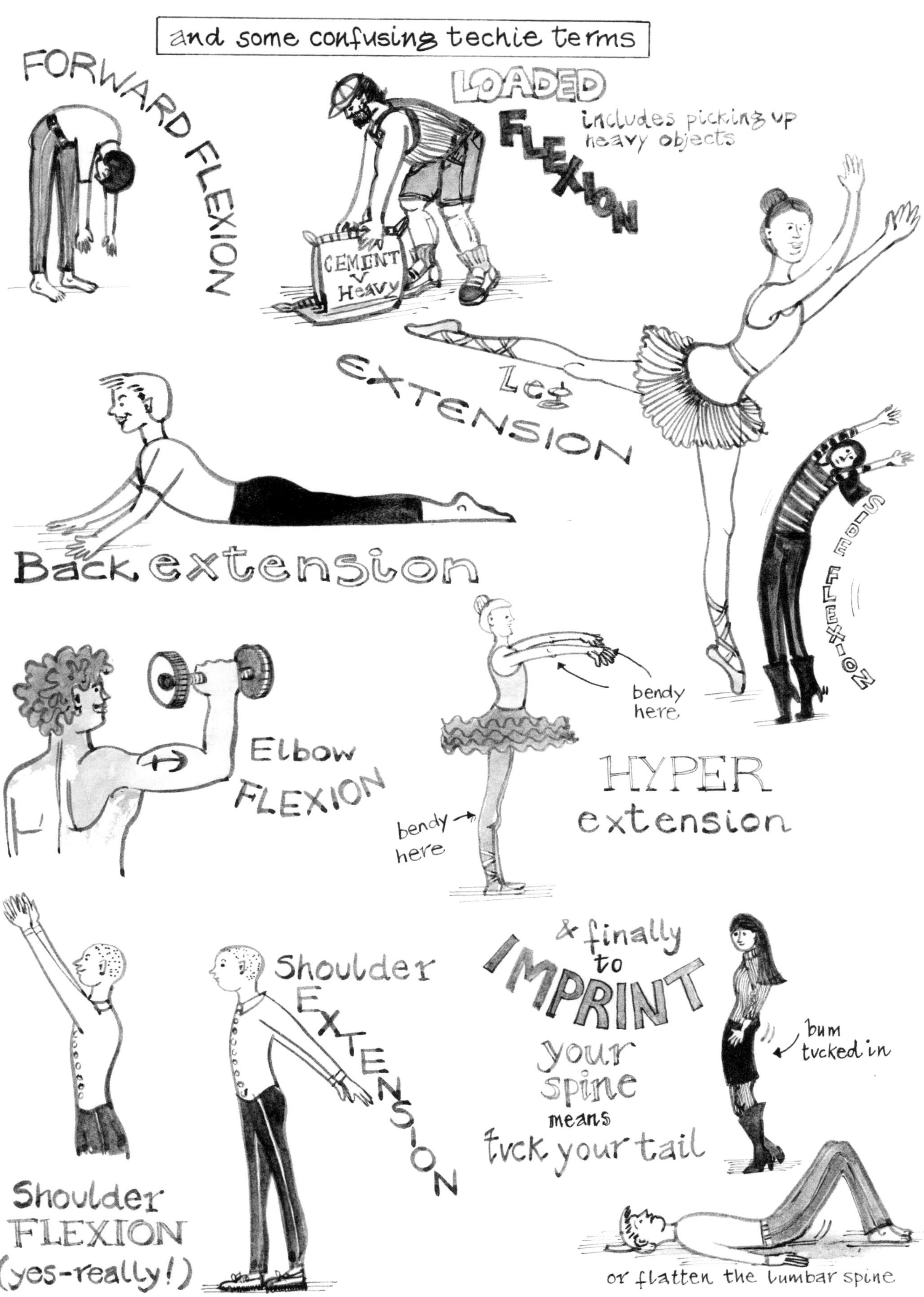
and some confusing techie terms
FORWARD FLEXION
LOADED FLEXION
includes picking up heavy objects
CEMENT V Heavy
Leg EXTENSION
Back extension
SIDE FLEXION
bendy here
HYPER extension
bendy here
Elbow FLEXION
Shoulder EXTENSION
Shoulder FLEXION (yes-really!)
& finally to IMPRINT your spine means tuck your tail
bum tucked in
or flatten the lumbar spine

STABILITY

IS ONE OF THE MOST IMPORTANT CONCEPTS IN PILATES & THE TERM CORE STABILITY HAS BEEN USED AS A UNIVERSAL PANACEA FOR ALL EXERCISE RELATED INJURIES & PROBLEMS.

Muscles around the joints work symbiotically: some are STABILISERS & some are MOVERS. When you are intending to move, set your tummy before moving your legs & set your shoulders before moving your arms. After a bit of practice this will become instinctive.

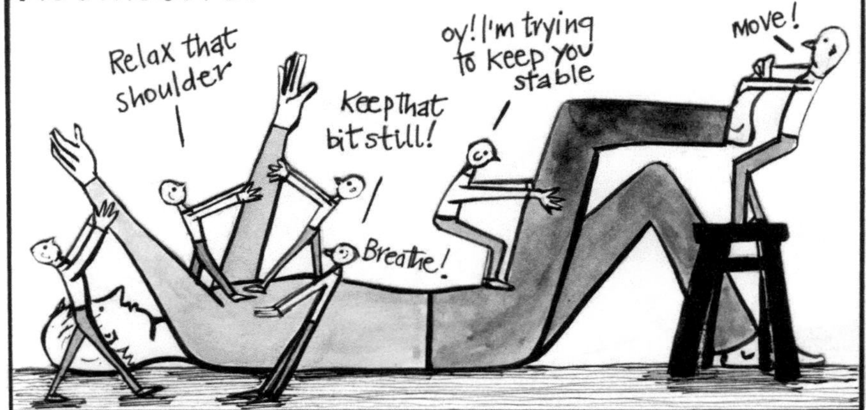

Good stability is the ability to keep one part of the body motionless while another part moves as freely as possible. The more solid the foundation is, the more efficient the movement can become.

Better Stability means better movement. Better movement means SAFER movement

TO MOVE THE ARMS EFFICIENTLY WE NEED SHOULDER (OR SCAPULAR) STABILITY. TO MOVE THE LEGS EFFICIENTLY, WE NEED SPINAL & PELVIC STABILITY & FOR THIS WE NEED STRONG ABDOMINALS.

TRY THE SPINAL STABILITY CHALLENGE BY FOLLOWING STEPS 1-6.

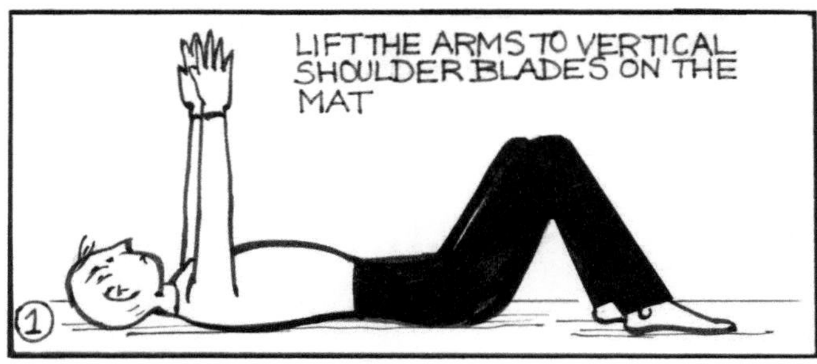

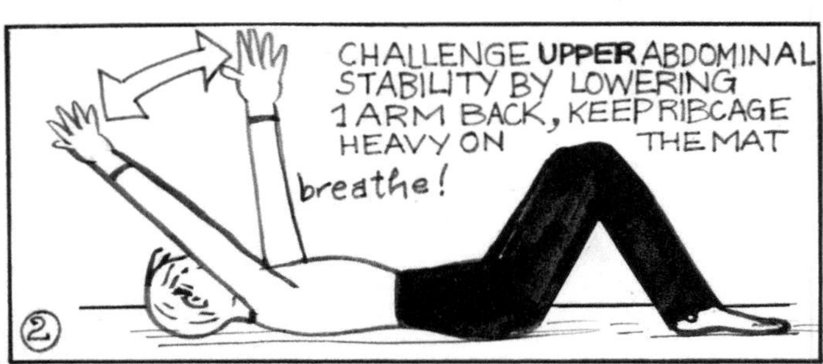

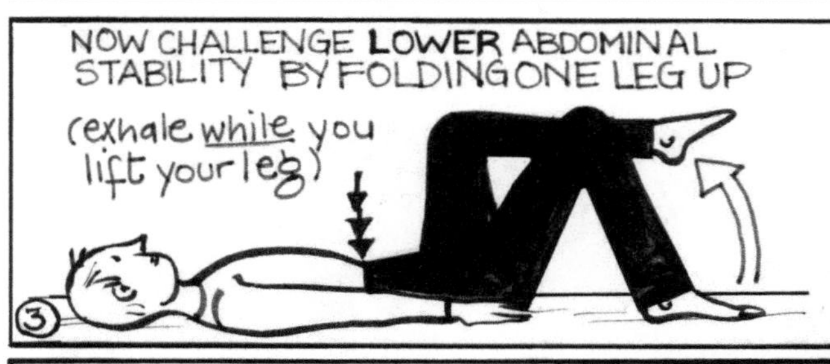

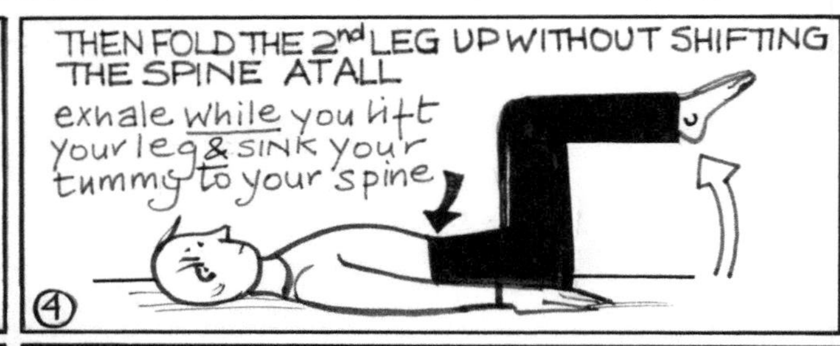

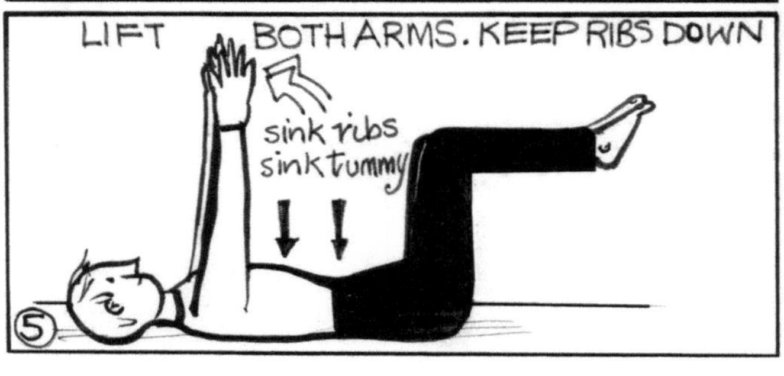

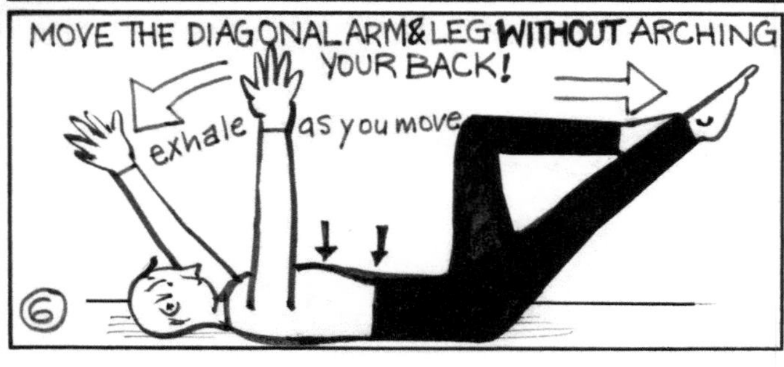

ASK CORA TO HELP YOU ANSWER YOUR PILATES QUESTIONS

Dear Cora, my teacher keeps telling me to work in neutral. I am too embarrassed to ask what this means. Are my leggings too garish?

Don't worry, she's not criticising your colour choices. 'Find neutral', 'Keep neutral', 'work in neutral' tend to be Pilates mantras. NEUTRAL is short for NEUTRAL SPINE or NEUTRAL PELVIS & means **not** flattening out the natural lumbar curve in the spine or tilting the pelvis. Contemporary Pilates encourages working in neutral as it keeps the back & abdominal muscles the correct length in order to support your spine when you stand up.

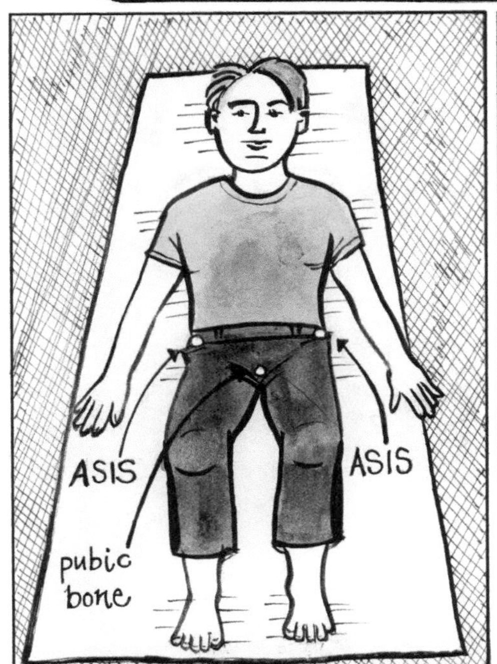

HOW TO FIND NEUTRAL PELVIS

Technically defined as being when the pubic bone & the two ASIS (hip bones) are in the same plane either in lying, standing or sitting. When you lie on your back the triangle between the ASIS & the pubic bones should be parallel to the floor. If you don't have a spirit level handy imagine balancing your drink on this tripod. (In this picture both SPINE & PELVIS are in neutral)

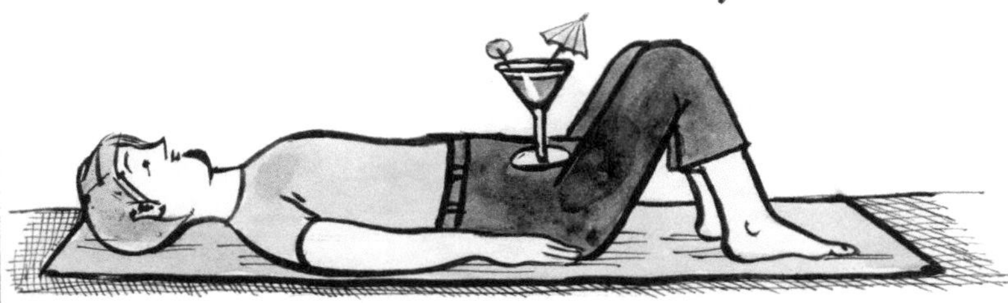

Don't spill the drink as you do an ab curl or a knee fold. (In this picture the PELVIS is in neutral but the SPINE is not.)

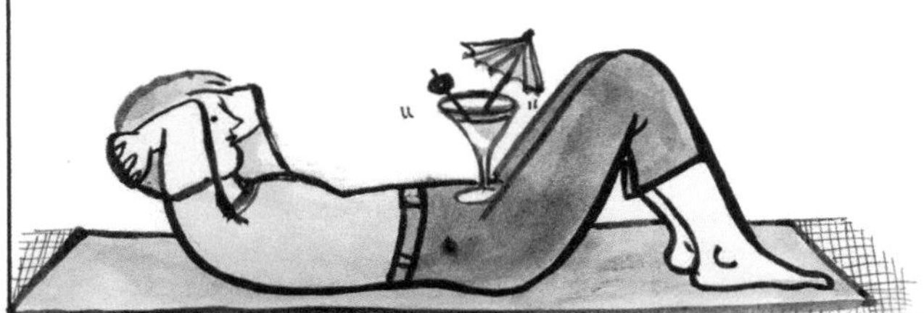

If the legs are straightened they place a greater load on the spine & you may need to IMPRINT (or tilt the pelvis) for support.

Neutral Pelvis is a relatively recent concept in Pilates as Jo originally taught his clients to tuck their tails under to flatten the back.

Top Tip

VARY your exercises.

Your body is designed to BEND, TWIST & STRETCH in different directions.

Don't allow it to get BORED

Section 2

The Essentials

Now it's time to roll out your mat and make yourself comfortable on the floor. Even doing ten minutes of Pilates exercise a day will make a big difference to your body and keep away those niggling aches and pains. Pick and mix or start with the exercises marked 1 and work your way to 3.

Try to find your deep Abdominals.

(they're the ones that will keep your lower back stable)

Teachers use lots of cues to encourage you to use the deep abdominal muscles instead of 'bracing' with your superficial muscles

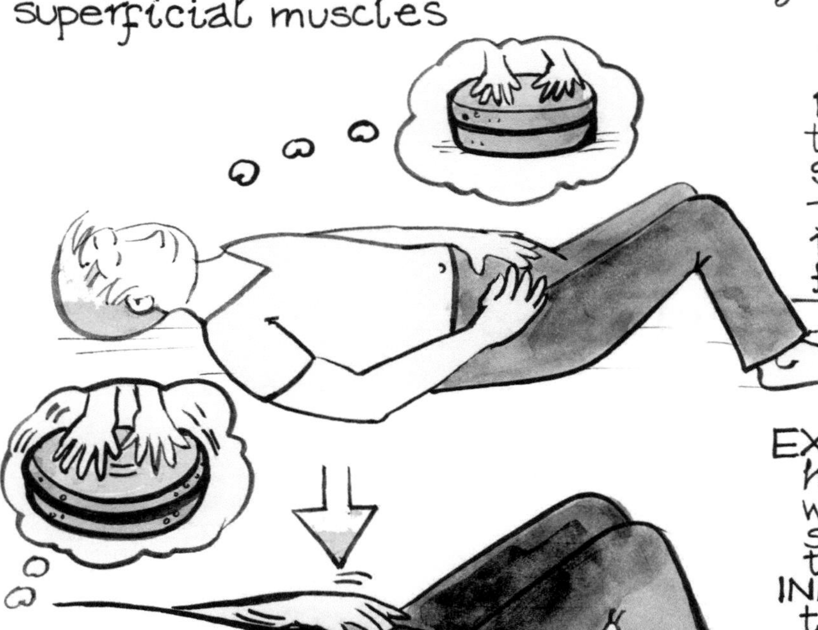

First you need to relax & let your tummy feel soft & spongy.

Take a couple of breaths in & out so it rises & falls.

EXHALE allowing your hands to sink down while your tummy sinks downwards towards your spine.

INHALE a sniff into the top of your lungs without your tummy popping up again.

Make sure your pelvis doesn't tilt as you do this!

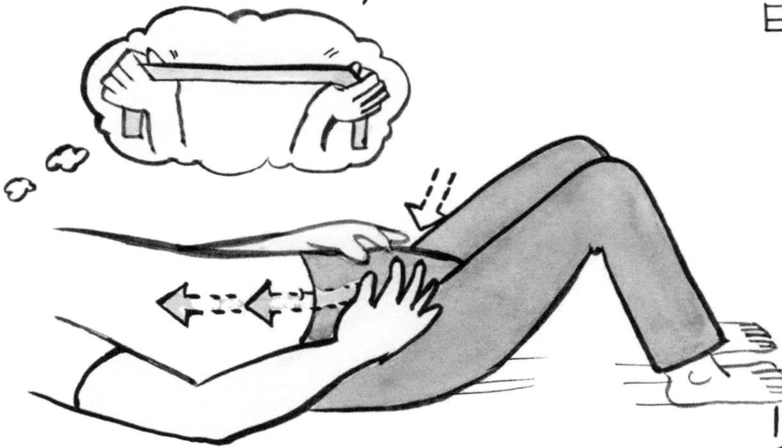

EXHALE to pull your tummy down even lower then try & pull it up under your ribs.

IMAGINE PULLING A RUBBER BAND UP FROM YOUR PUBIC BONE, DEEP INSIDE YOU & UNDER YOUR RIBCAGE

This will be enough to keep your back stable.

INHALE (sniff) again & still don't "pop" the abdominals.

EXHALE S-L-O-W-L-Y to release the tension

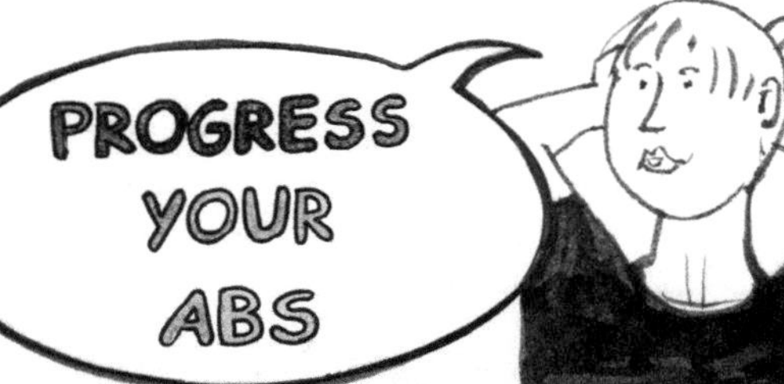

IF YOU'VE MASTERED THE STABILITY CHALLENGE, IT'S TIME TO ADD UPPER BODY FLEXION. FLEXING THE HEAD & SHOULDERS FORWARD WHILE KEEPING THE REST OF THE SPINE IN A NATURAL OR NEUTRAL POSITION WORKS THE UPPER ABDOMINAL MUSCLES. **LIFT YOUR LEGS & YOU WORK EVEN HARDER**

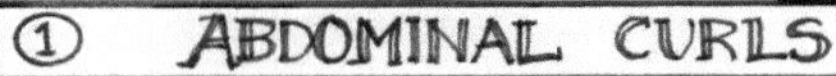

① ABDOMINAL CURLS — REPEAT 4–6

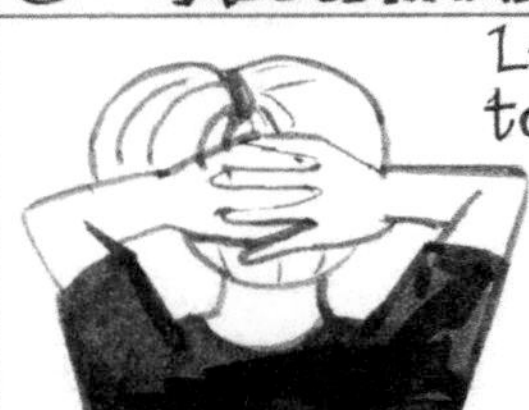

Exhale: curl forward

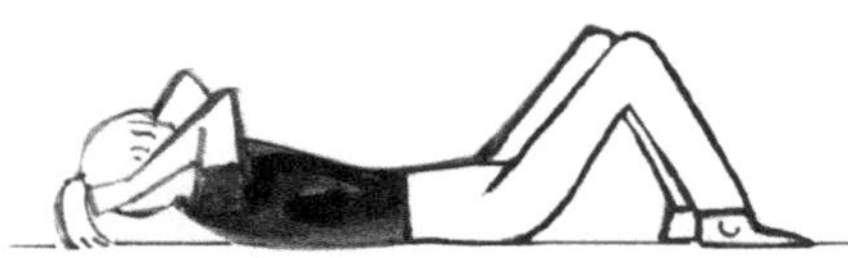

Inhale: hold position
Exhale: roll down slowly.

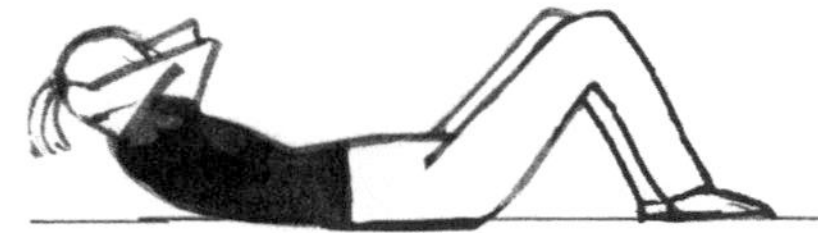

② TWIST & PULSES — REPEAT BOTH SIDES

Exhale: curl forward

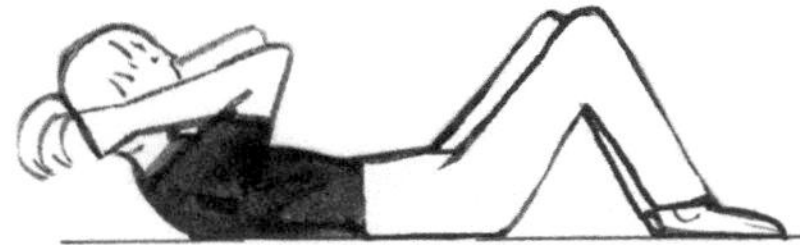

Slide one hand to opposite thigh – pulse across ×4

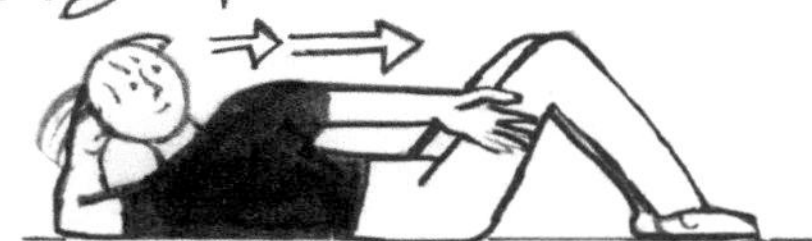

Repeat other side
Exhale & Inhale to pulse

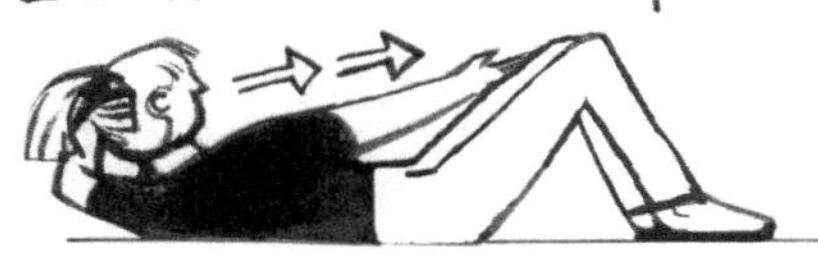

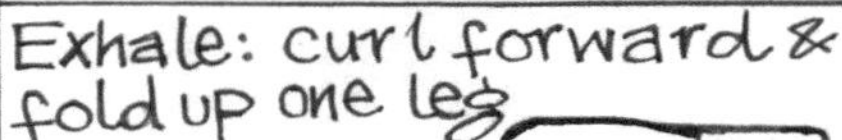

② ABDOMINAL CURLS & KNEE FOLDS — REPEAT 6–8

Exhale: curl forward & fold up one leg

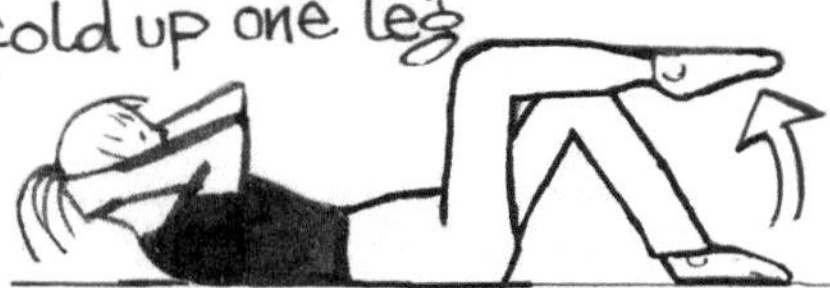

Inhale: deepen curl
Exhale: slowly lower leg

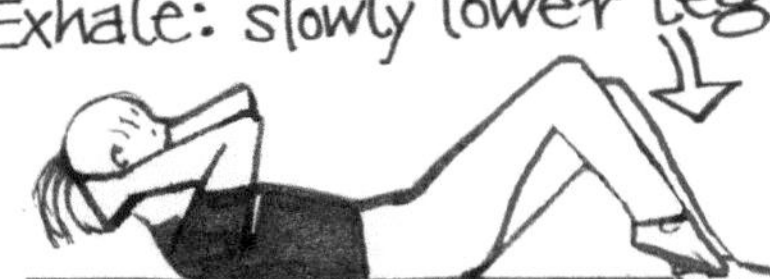

Roll down & repeat other leg

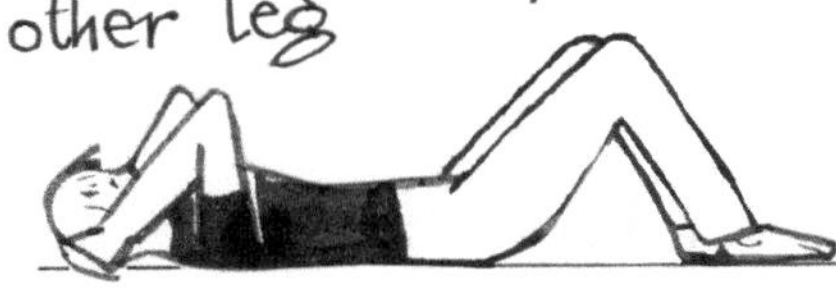

③ TOE TAPS — REPEAT 3 SETS

Exhale: curl forward

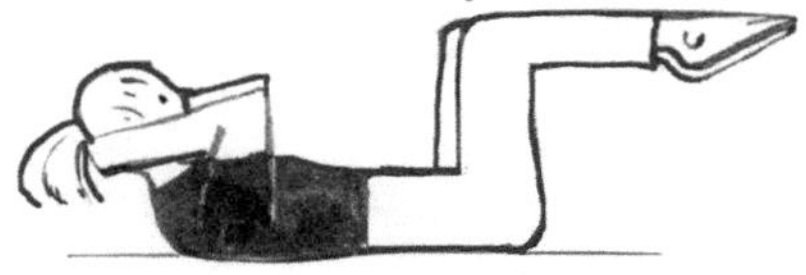

Inhale & Exhale: tap feet

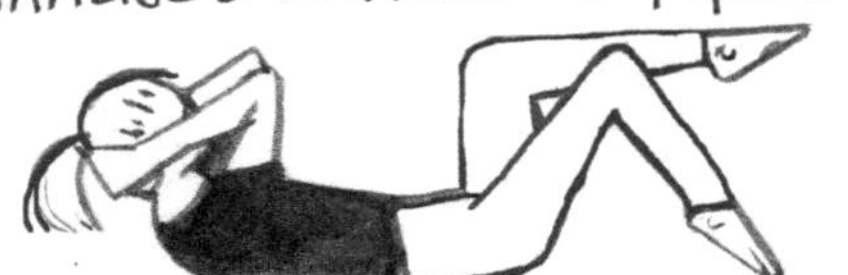

Alternate legs

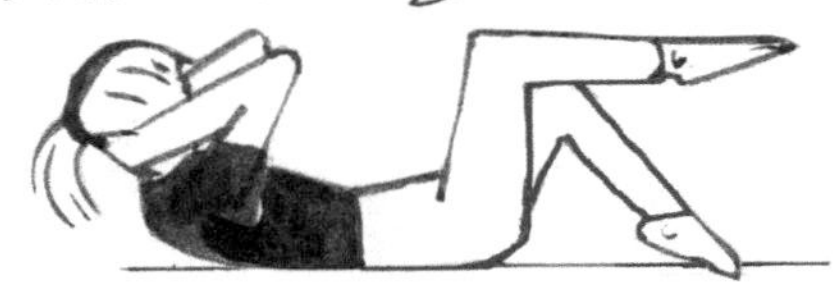

③ SINGLE LEG STRETCH — REPEAT 6–8 PER LEG

Exhale: curl forward

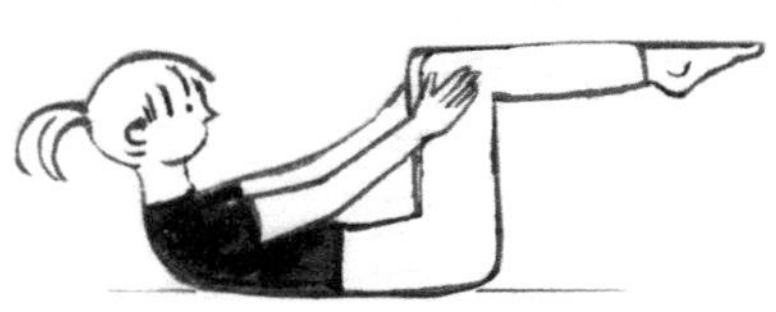

Bend one leg & lengthen the other

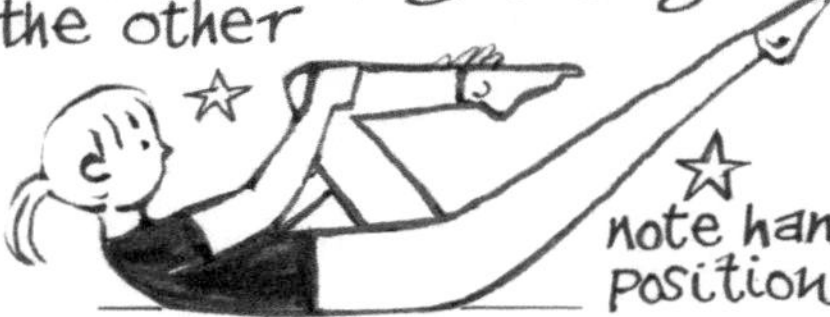

Exhale & Inhale: swop legs dynamically

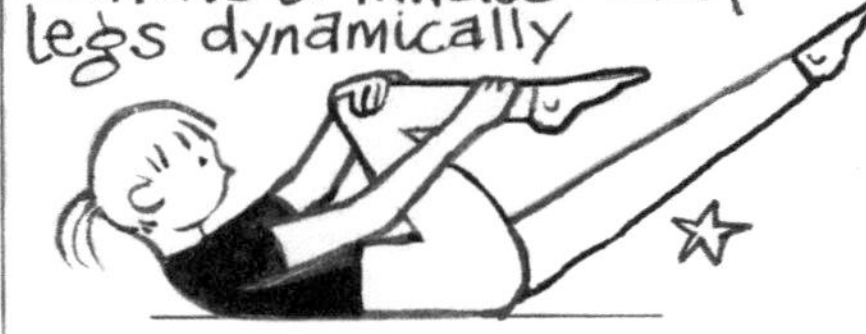

③ THE ROCKER — REPEAT 6–8 ROCKS

Curl forward. Exhale to twist

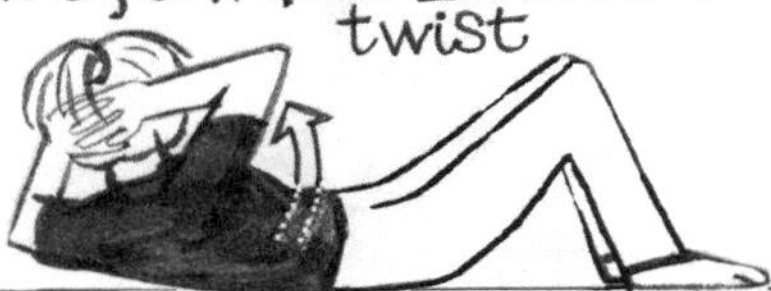

Inhale: Rock to centre. Keep curled forward

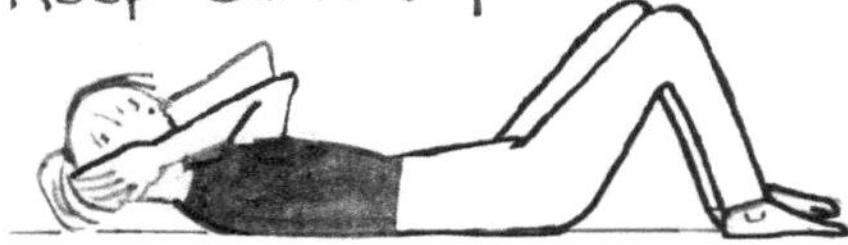

Exhale: twist to other side

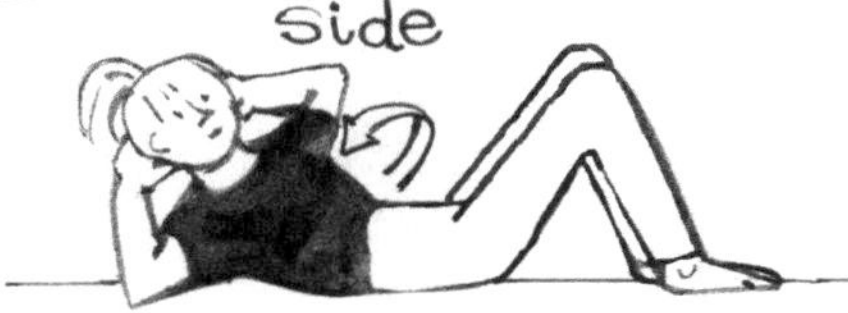

③ DOUBLE LEG GLIDE — REPEAT 6

Hold abdominal curl

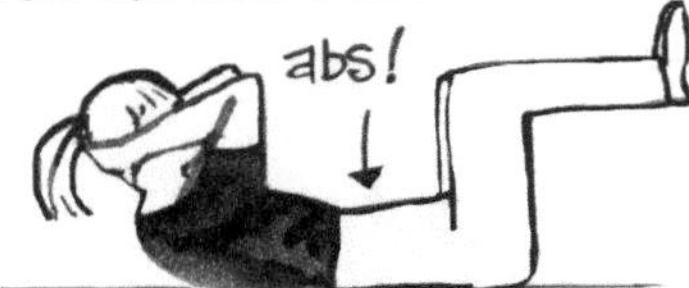

Curl higher & glide legs

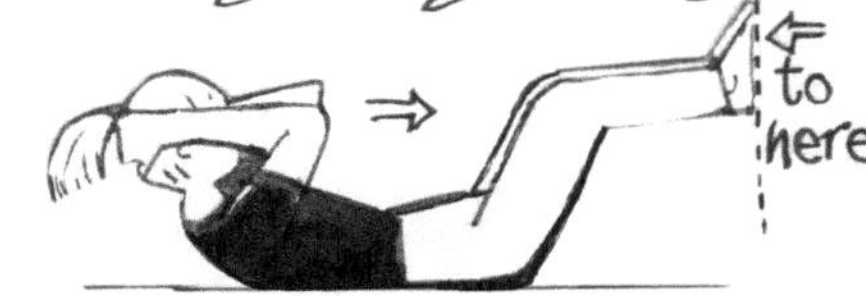

Glide legs back so ribs drop back a little

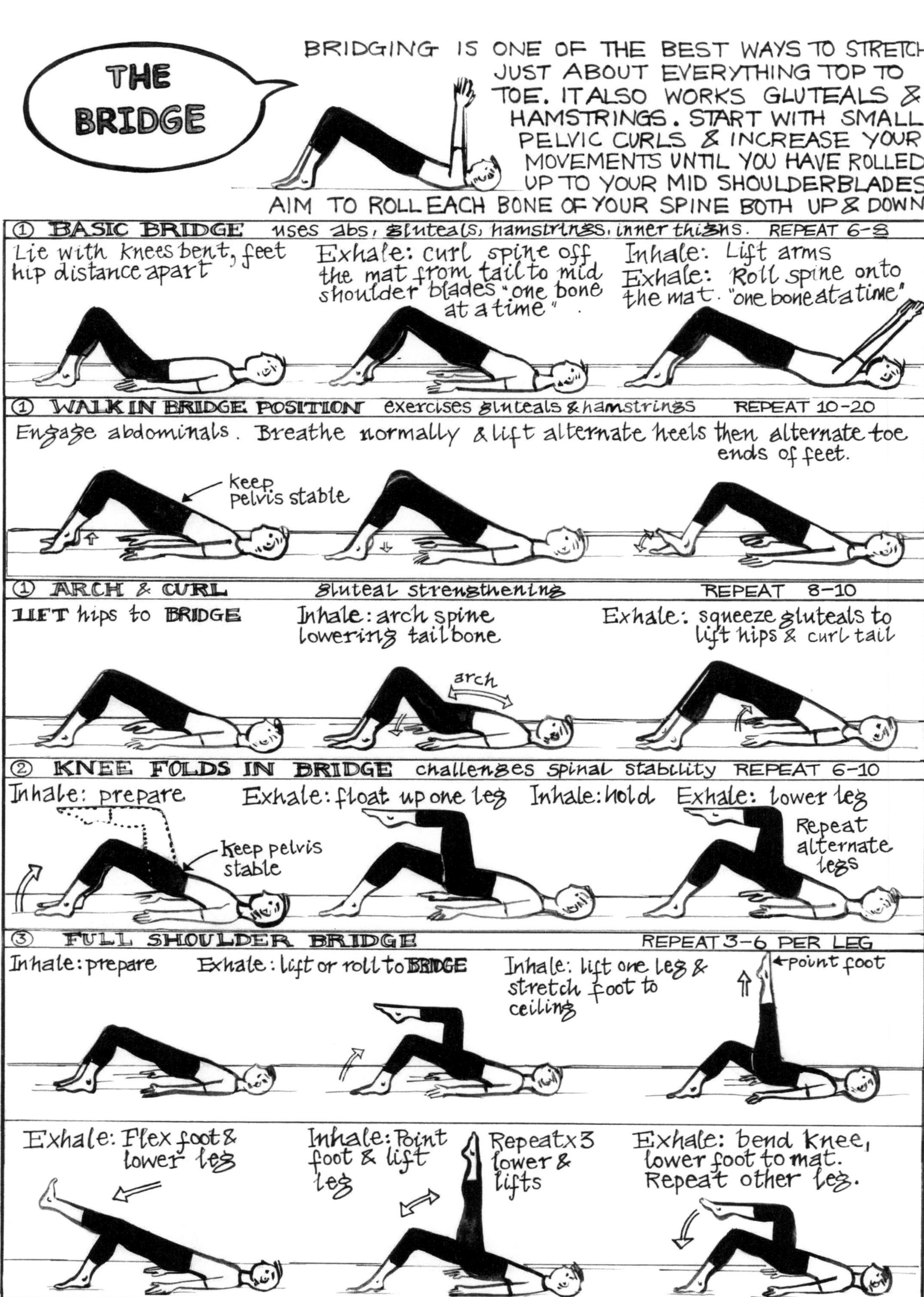
THE BRIDGE
BRIDGING IS ONE OF THE BEST WAYS TO STRETCH JUST ABOUT EVERYTHING TOP TO TOE. IT ALSO WORKS GLUTEALS & HAMSTRINGS. START WITH SMALL PELVIC CURLS & INCREASE YOUR MOVEMENTS UNTIL YOU HAVE ROLLED UP TO YOUR MID SHOULDERBLADES. AIM TO ROLL EACH BONE OF YOUR SPINE BOTH UP & DOWN.
① BASIC BRIDGE uses abs, gluteals, hamstrings, inner thighs. REPEAT 6-8
Lie with knees bent, feet hip distance apart
Exhale: curl spine off the mat from tail to mid shoulder blades "one bone at a time".
Inhale: Lift arms
Exhale: Roll spine onto the mat. "one bone at a time"
① WALK IN BRIDGE POSITION exercises gluteals & hamstrings REPEAT 10-20
Engage abdominals. Breathe normally & lift alternate heels then alternate toe ends of feet.
keep pelvis stable
① ARCH & CURL gluteal strengthening REPEAT 8-10
LIFT hips to BRIDGE
Inhale: arch spine lowering tail bone
arch
Exhale: squeeze gluteals to lift hips & curl tail
② KNEE FOLDS IN BRIDGE challenges spinal stability REPEAT 6-10
Inhale: prepare
Keep pelvis stable
Exhale: float up one leg
Inhale: hold
Exhale: lower leg
Repeat alternate legs
③ FULL SHOULDER BRIDGE REPEAT 3-6 PER LEG
Inhale: prepare
Exhale: lift or roll to BRIDGE
Inhale: lift one leg & stretch foot to ceiling
point foot
Exhale: Flex foot & lower leg
Inhale: Point foot & lift leg
Repeat x3 lower & lifts
Exhale: bend knee, lower foot to mat. Repeat other leg.

ALL BUTTS

Strengthen your backside & balance your hips

LYING ON ONE SIDE OR KNEELING ON ALL FOURS CAN OFTEN MAKE IT EASIER TO EXERCISE IN ORDER TO MOBILISE THE HIPS, STRENGTHEN THE GLUTEALS & IMPROVE SPINAL STABILITY.
STIFF & UNBALANCED HIP MUSCLES CAN CAUSE PAIN IN THE BACK, LEGS & IN THE HIPS THEMSELVES.

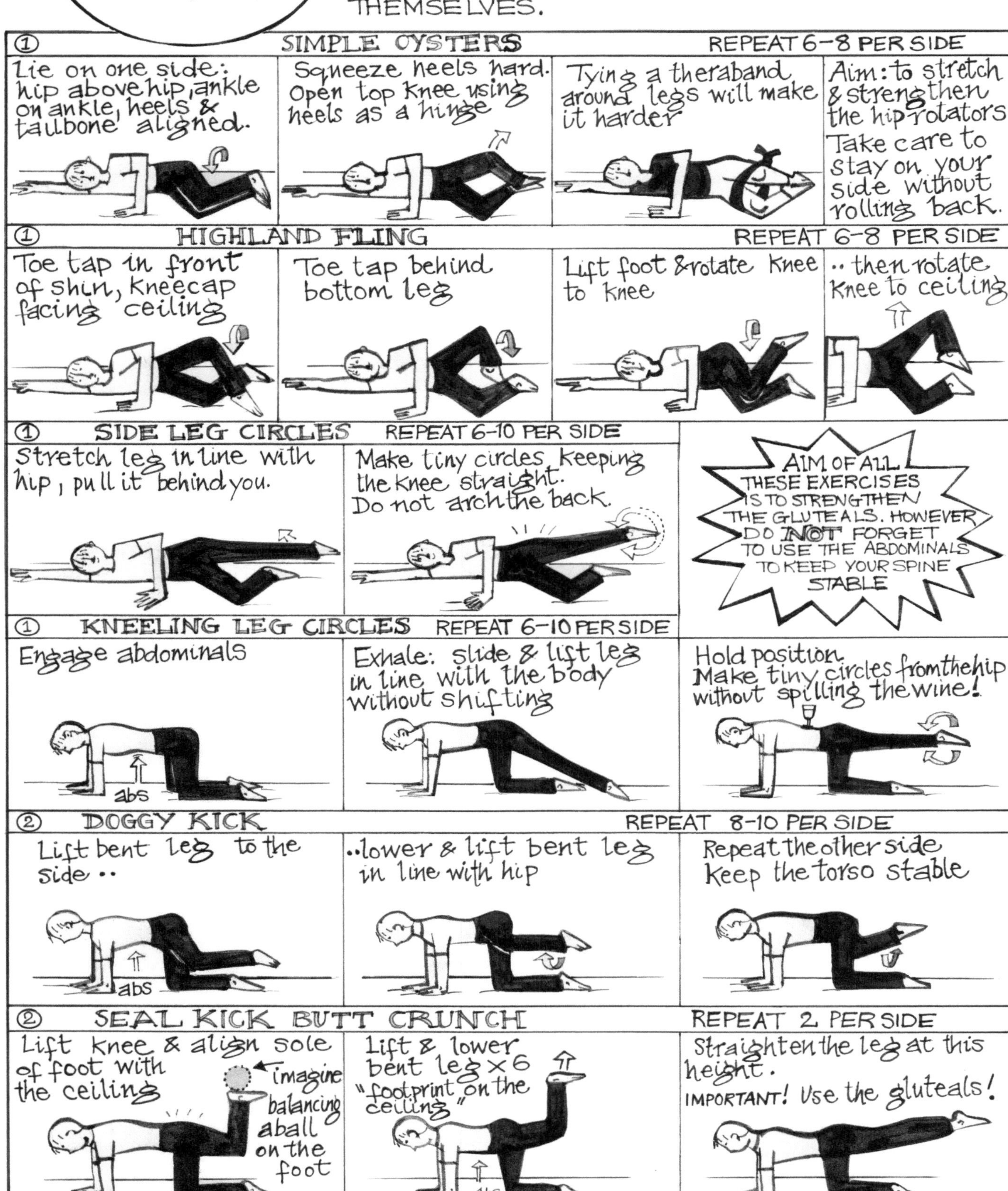

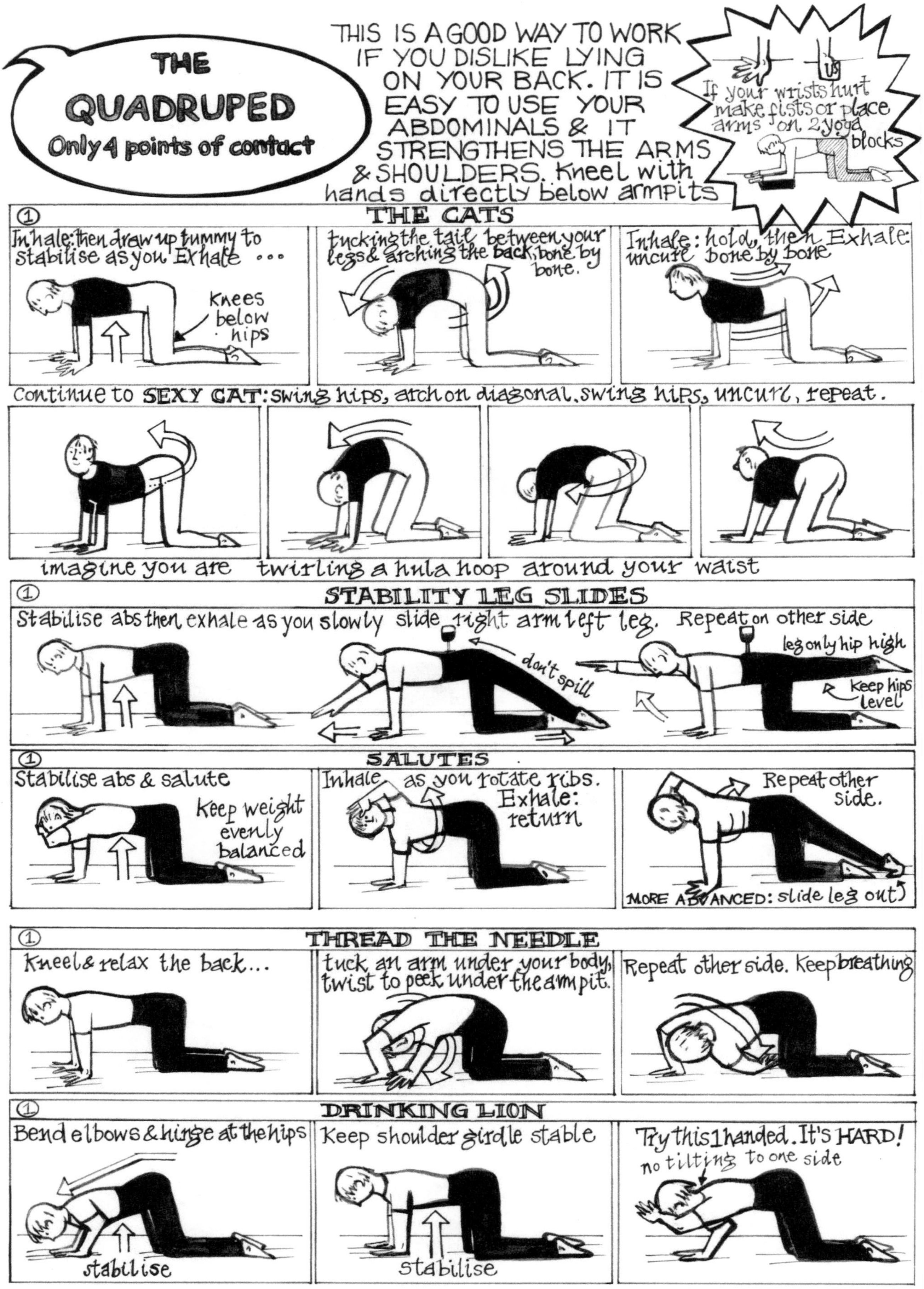

THE QUADRUPED

Only 4 points of contact

THIS IS A GOOD WAY TO WORK IF YOU DISLIKE LYING ON YOUR BACK. IT IS EASY TO USE YOUR ABDOMINALS & IT STRENGTHENS THE ARMS & SHOULDERS. Kneel with hands directly below armpits

If your wrists hurt make fists or place arms on 2 yoga blocks

① THE CATS

Inhale: then draw up tummy to stabilise as you Exhale ...

Knees below hips

tucking the tail between your legs & arching the back, bone by bone.

Inhale: hold, then Exhale: uncurl bone by bone

Continue to **SEXY CAT**: swing hips, arch on diagonal, swing hips, uncurl, repeat.

imagine you are twirling a hula hoop around your waist

① STABILITY LEG SLIDES

Stabilise abs then exhale as you slowly slide right arm left leg. Repeat on other side

don't spill

leg only hip high

keep hips level

① SALUTES

Stabilise abs & salute

Keep weight evenly balanced

Inhale as you rotate ribs. Exhale: return

Repeat other side.

MORE ADVANCED: slide leg out

① THREAD THE NEEDLE

Kneel & relax the back...

tuck an arm under your body, twist to peek under the armpit.

Repeat other side. Keep breathing

① DRINKING LION

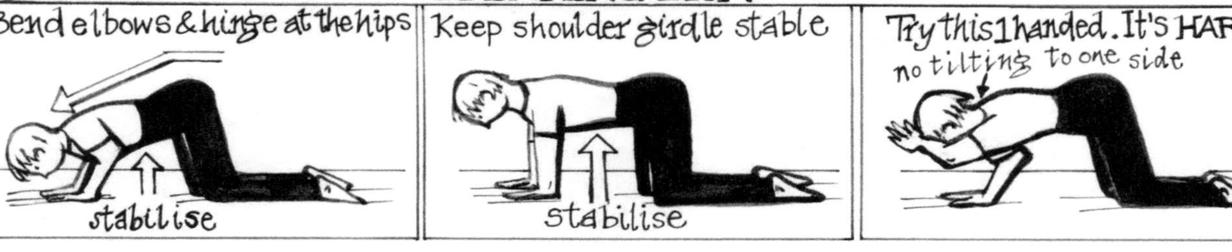

SIDEWAYS
A safe way to use your abdominals & gluteals together
oooh
these are adductors
so are these

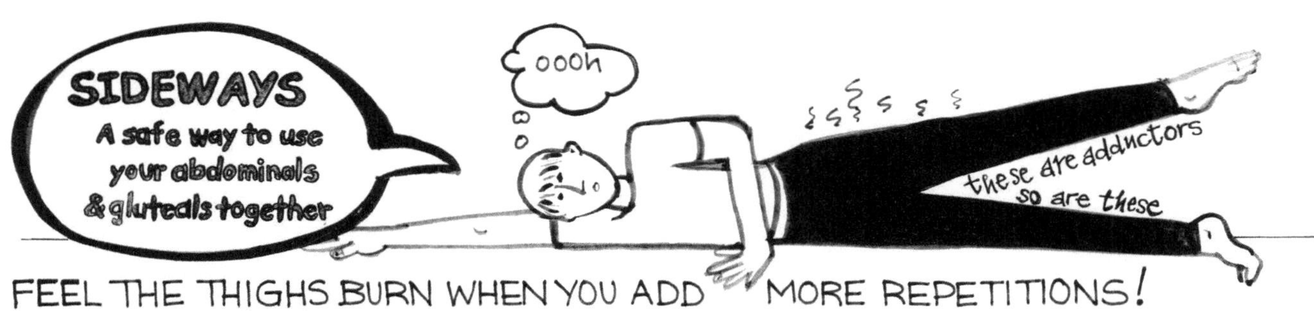

FEEL THE THIGHS BURN WHEN YOU ADD MORE REPETITIONS!

① SINGLE LEG LIFT 1 — REPEAT 6-8 ON BOTH SIDES

Lie on your side. Reach out with the legs, then draw them slightly forward so the back won't arch.

Inhale: to lift top leg, point foot

Exhale: to lower leg with flexed foot

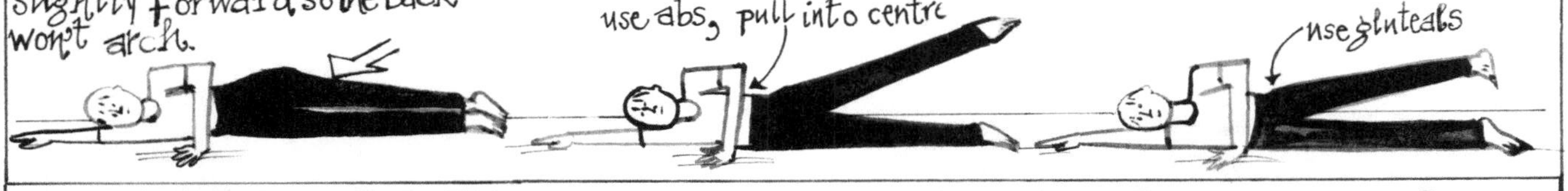
use abs, pull into centre
use gluteals

① SINGLE LEG LIFT 2 — REPEAT 6-8 ON BOTH SIDES

Inhale: to lift top leg .... & Inhaling: lift lower leg in point

Exhale: lower both legs with flexed feet

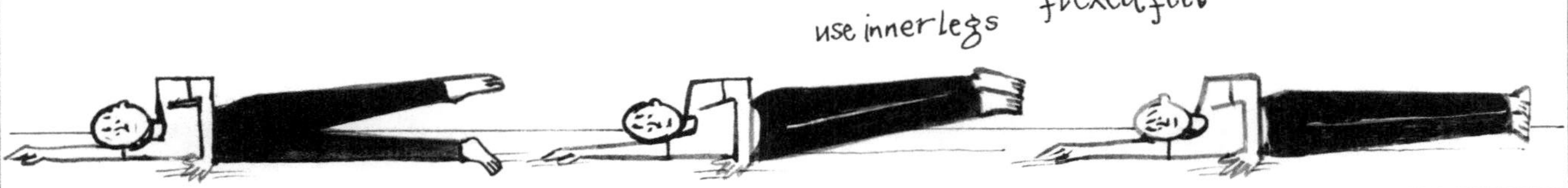
use inner legs

② BEATS — REPEAT 10-20 BEATS PER SIDE

Hover both legs. Open both legs, squeeze together. Increase speed to challenge

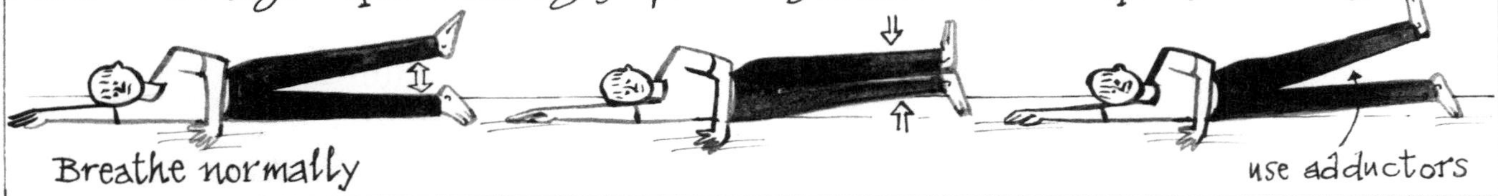
Breathe normally
use adductors

③ DOUBLE LEG LIFT — REPEAT 6-8 ON BOTH SIDES

Exhale: to lift both legs

slide hand toward knee, point feet. Inhale: to lower legs, flex feet

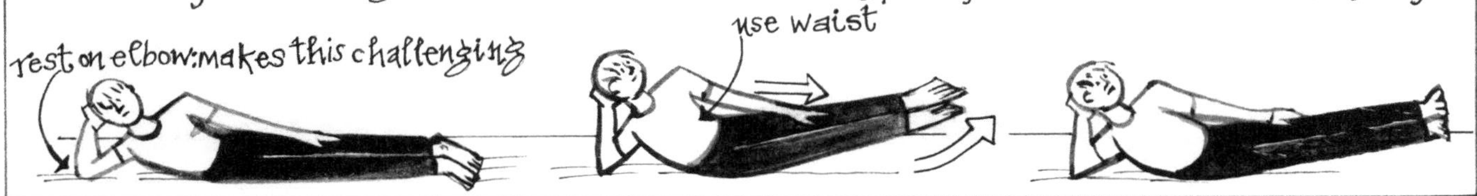
rest on elbow: makes this challenging
use waist

③ SIDE KICK LYING — REPEAT 6-8 ON BOTH SIDES

Lift top leg in line with hip

Inhale: sweep leg behind you, point foot

Exhale: sweep leg forward, flex foot to activate back of leg

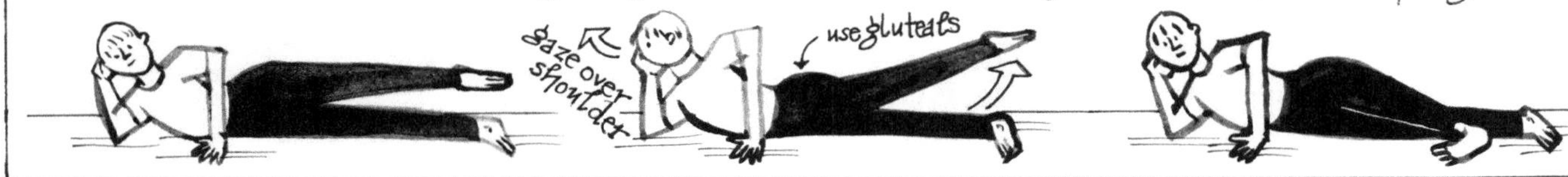
gaze over shoulder
use gluteals

③ SCISSORS — REPEAT 10-12 SCISSORS PER SIDE

Hover both legs: hip height

Scissor legs back & forward in opposition Inhaling & Exhaling

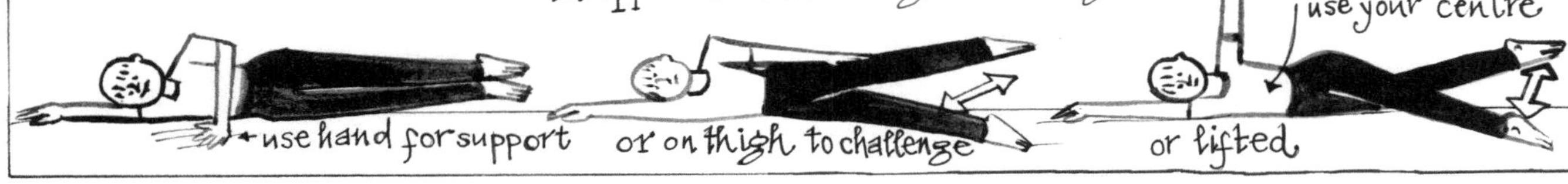
use your centre
use hand for support
or on thigh to challenge
or lifted

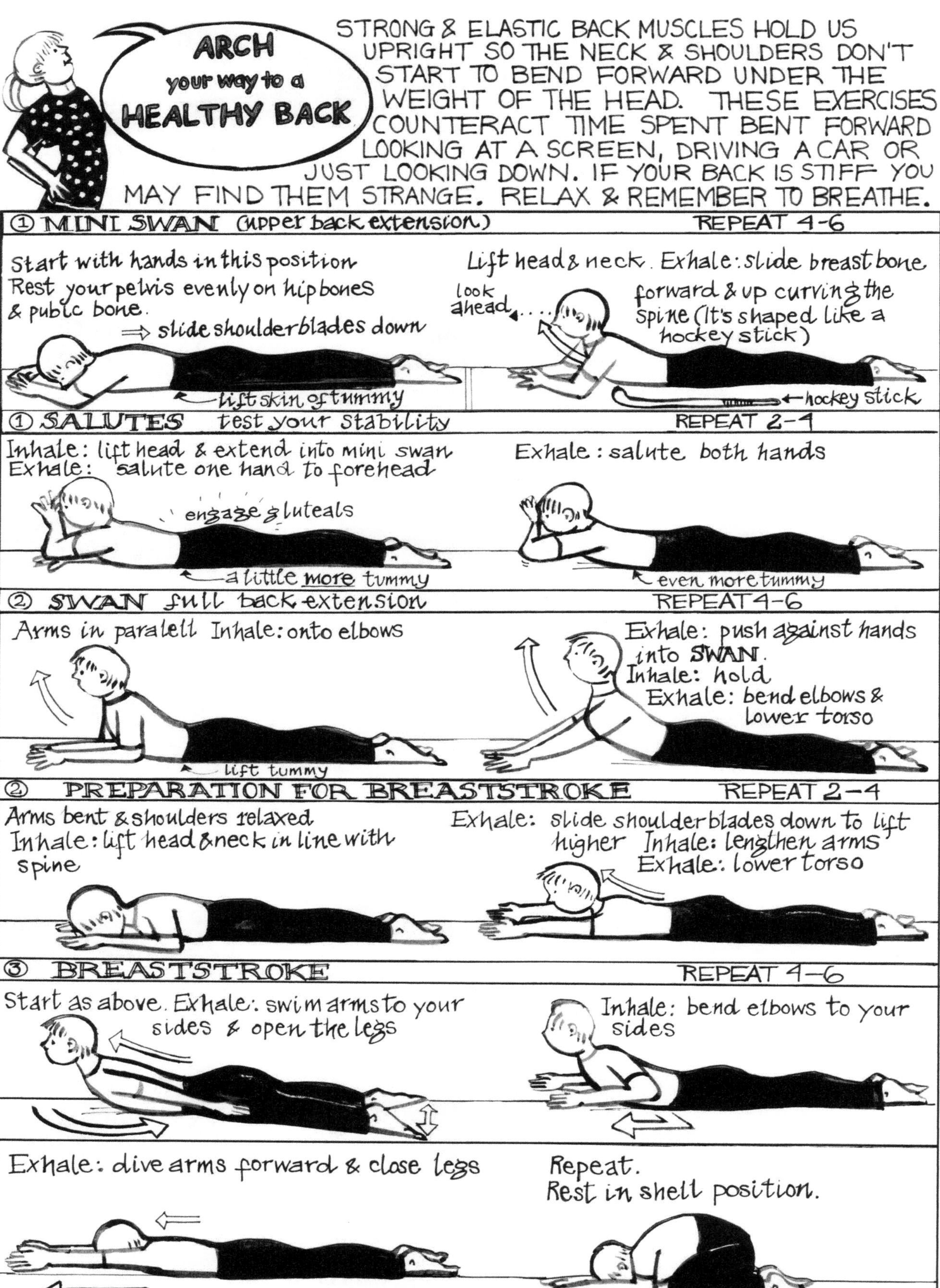
ARCH your way to a HEALTHY BACK
STRONG & ELASTIC BACK MUSCLES HOLD US UPRIGHT SO THE NECK & SHOULDERS DON'T START TO BEND FORWARD UNDER THE WEIGHT OF THE HEAD. THESE EXERCISES COUNTERACT TIME SPENT BENT FORWARD LOOKING AT A SCREEN, DRIVING A CAR OR JUST LOOKING DOWN. IF YOUR BACK IS STIFF YOU MAY FIND THEM STRANGE. RELAX & REMEMBER TO BREATHE.
① MINI SWAN (upper back extension)
REPEAT 4-6
Start with hands in this position
Rest your pelvis evenly on hip bones & pubic bone.
⇒ slide shoulderblades down
← lift skin of tummy
Lift head & neck. Exhale: slide breast bone forward & up curving the spine (It's shaped like a hockey stick)
look ahead
← hockey stick
① SALUTES test your stability
REPEAT 2-4
Inhale: lift head & extend into mini swan
Exhale: salute one hand to forehead
engage gluteals
← a little more tummy
Exhale: salute both hands
← even more tummy
② SWAN full back extension
REPEAT 4-6
Arms in paralell Inhale: onto elbows
← lift tummy
Exhale: push against hands into SWAN.
Inhale: hold
Exhale: bend elbows & lower torso
② PREPARATION FOR BREASTSTROKE
REPEAT 2-4
Arms bent & shoulders relaxed
Inhale: lift head & neck in line with spine
Exhale: slide shoulderblades down to lift higher Inhale: lengthen arms
Exhale: lower torso
③ BREASTSTROKE
REPEAT 4-6
Start as above. Exhale: swim arms to your sides & open the legs
Inhale: bend elbows to your sides
Exhale: dive arms forward & close legs
Repeat.
Rest in shell position.

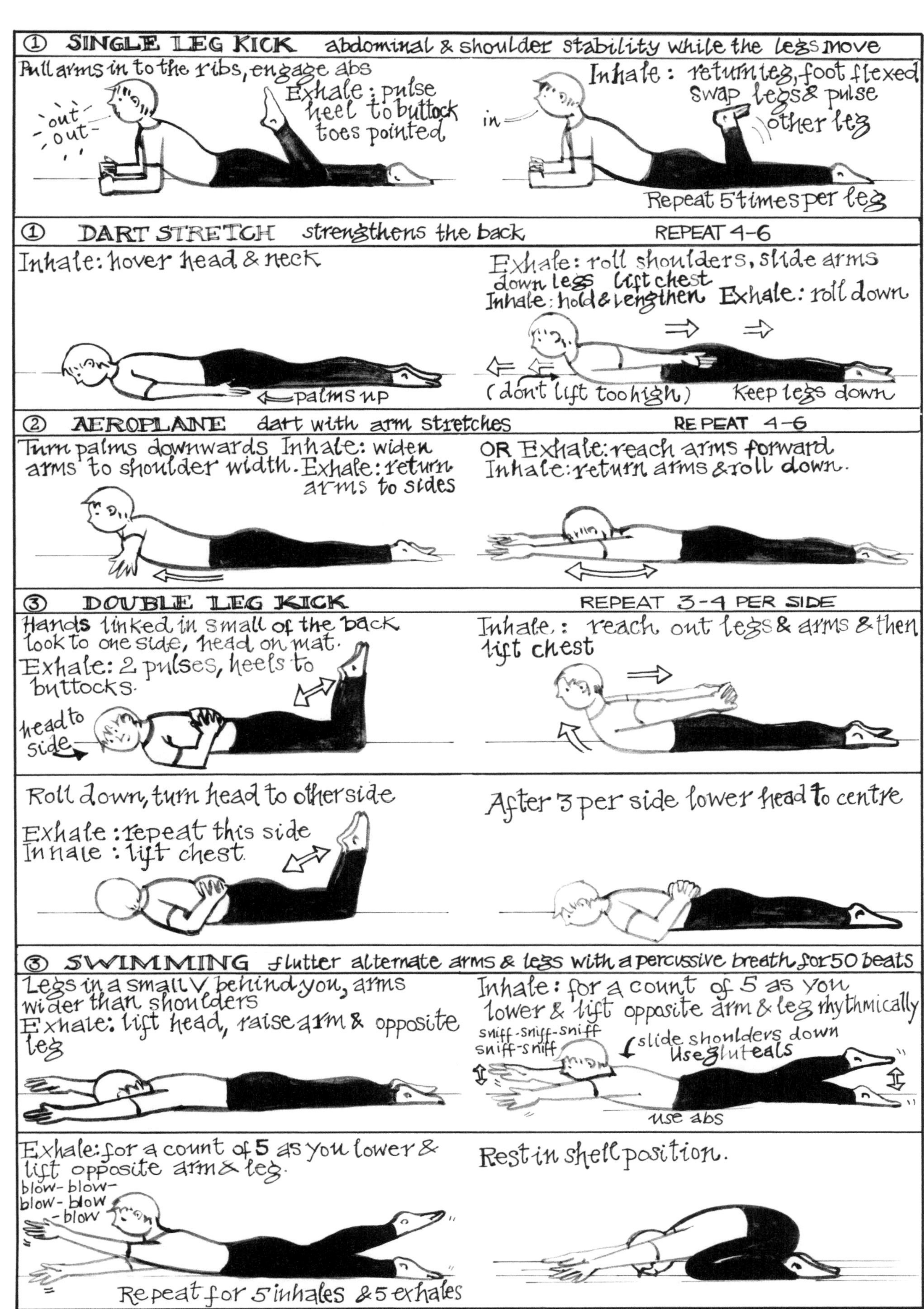
① SINGLE LEG KICK abdominal & shoulder stability while the legs move
Pull arms in to the ribs, engage abs
Exhale: pulse heel to buttock toes pointed
out out
in
Inhale: return leg, foot flexed swap legs & pulse other leg
Repeat 5 times per leg
① DART STRETCH strengthens the back REPEAT 4-6
Inhale: hover head & neck
palms up
Exhale: roll shoulders, slide arms down legs lift chest
Inhale: hold & lengthen Exhale: roll down
(don't lift too high)
Keep legs down
② AEROPLANE dart with arm stretches REPEAT 4-6
Turn palms downwards Inhale: widen arms to shoulder width. Exhale: return arms to sides
OR Exhale: reach arms forward Inhale: return arms & roll down.
③ DOUBLE LEG KICK REPEAT 3-4 PER SIDE
Hands linked in small of the back look to one side, head on mat.
Exhale: 2 pulses, heels to buttocks.
head to side
Inhale: reach out legs & arms & then lift chest
Roll down, turn head to other side
Exhale: repeat this side
Inhale: lift chest
After 3 per side lower head to centre
③ SWIMMING flutter alternate arms & legs with a percussive breath for 50 beats
Legs in a small V behind you, arms wider than shoulders
Exhale: lift head, raise arm & opposite leg
Inhale: for a count of 5 as you lower & lift opposite arm & leg rhythmically
sniff-sniff-sniff sniff-sniff
slide shoulders down
Use gluteals
use abs
Exhale: for a count of 5 as you lower & lift opposite arm & leg.
blow-blow-blow-blow-blow
Repeat for 5 inhales & 5 exhales
Rest in shell position.

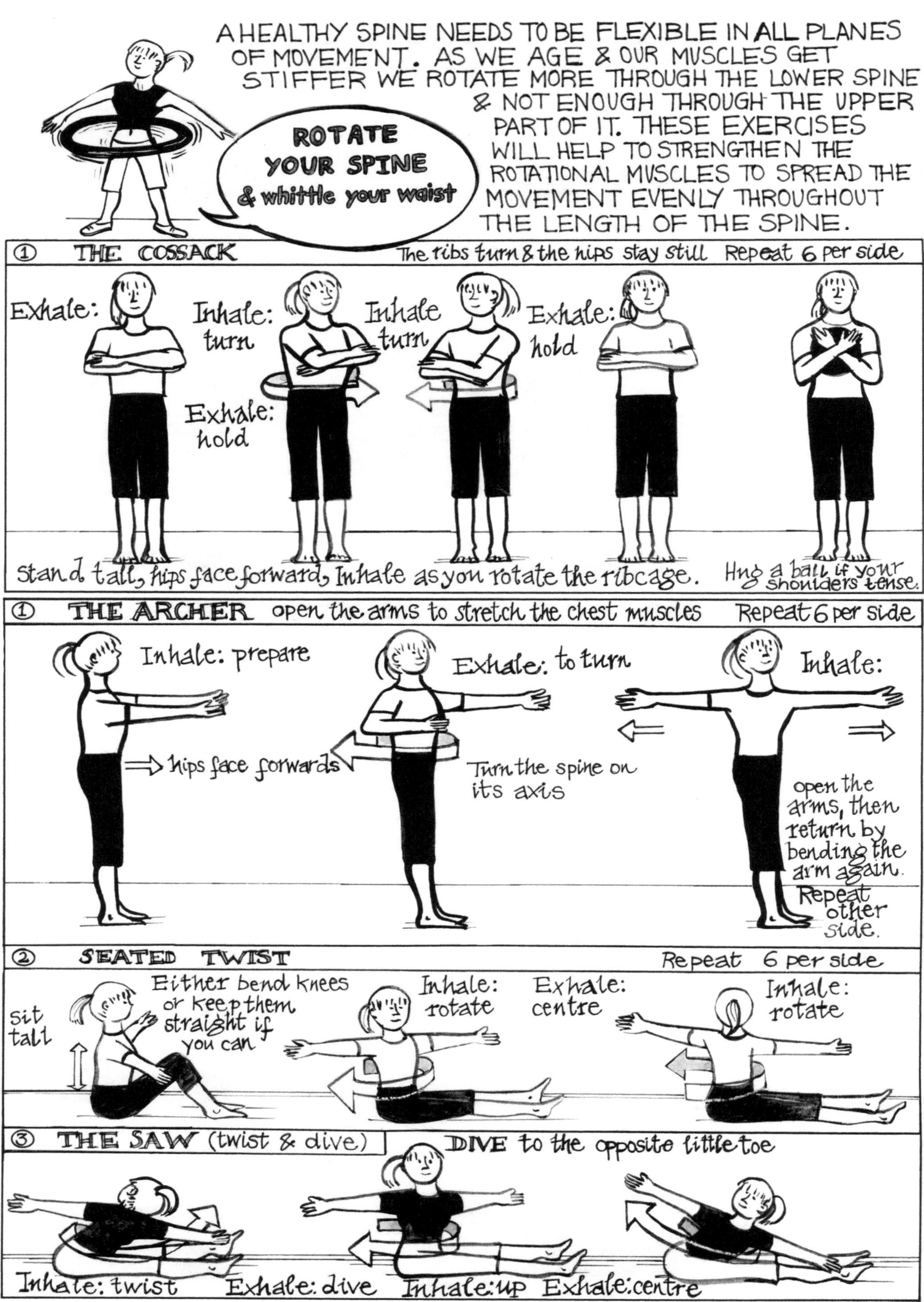
A HEALTHY SPINE NEEDS TO BE FLEXIBLE IN ALL PLANES OF MOVEMENT. AS WE AGE & OUR MUSCLES GET STIFFER WE ROTATE MORE THROUGH THE LOWER SPINE & NOT ENOUGH THROUGH THE UPPER PART OF IT. THESE EXERCISES WILL HELP TO STRENGTHEN THE ROTATIONAL MUSCLES TO SPREAD THE MOVEMENT EVENLY THROUGHOUT THE LENGTH OF THE SPINE.
ROTATE YOUR SPINE
& whittle your waist
① THE COSSACK
The ribs turn & the hips stay still
Repeat 6 per side
Exhale:
Inhale: turn
Exhale: hold
Inhale turn
Exhale: hold
Stand tall, hips face forward, Inhale as you rotate the ribcage.
Hug a ball if your shoulders tense.
① THE ARCHER
open the arms to stretch the chest muscles
Repeat 6 per side
Inhale: prepare
hips face forwards
Exhale: to turn
Turn the spine on its axis
Inhale:
open the arms, then return by bending the arm again. Repeat other side.
② SEATED TWIST
Repeat 6 per side
sit tall
Either bend knees or keep them straight if you can
Inhale: rotate
Exhale: centre
Inhale: rotate
③ THE SAW (twist & dive)
DIVE to the opposite little toe
Inhale: twist
Exhale: dive
Inhale: up
Exhale: centre

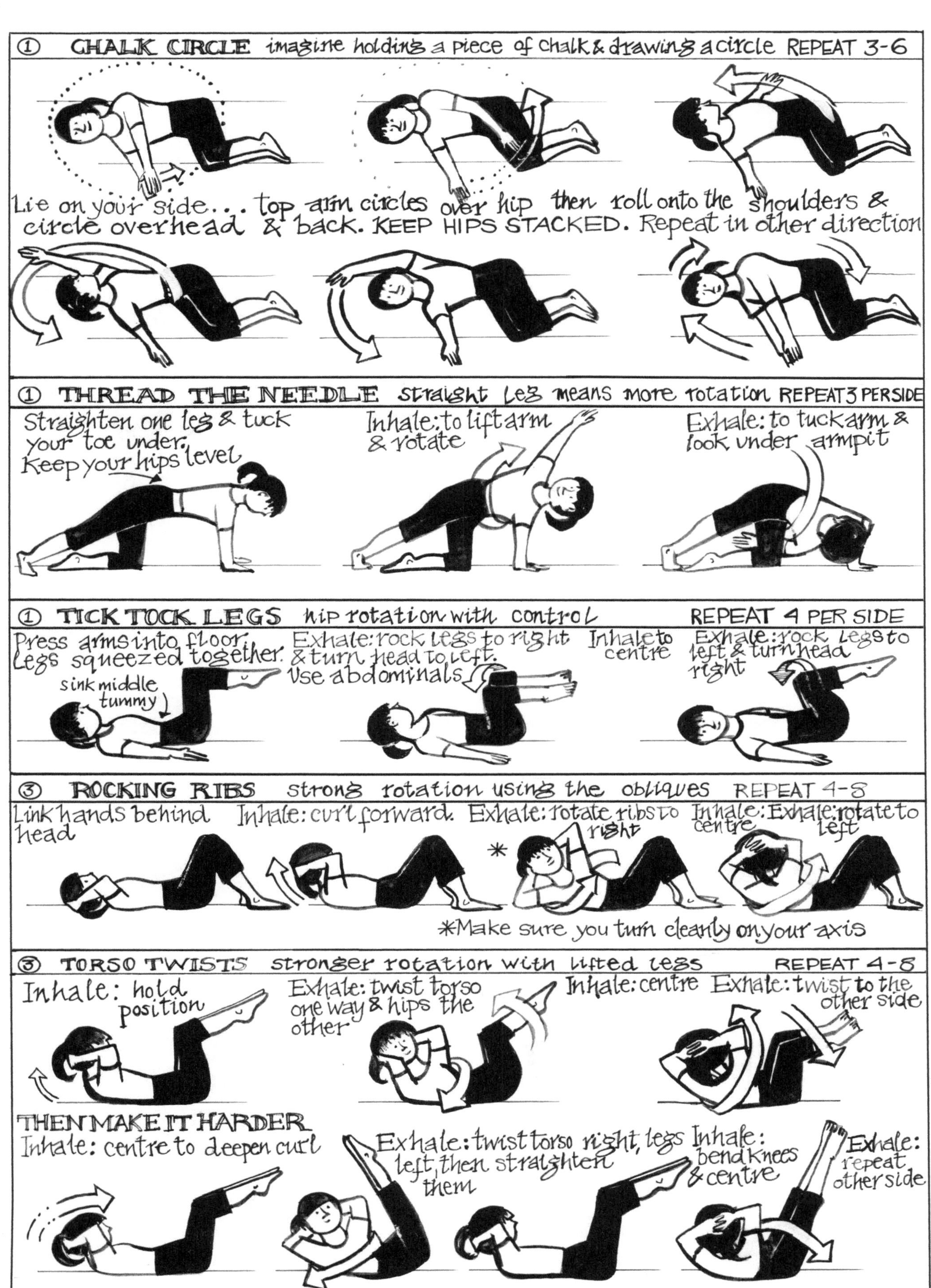
① CHALK CIRCLE imagine holding a piece of chalk & drawing a circle REPEAT 3-6
Lie on your side... top arm circles over hip then roll onto the shoulders & circle overhead & back. KEEP HIPS STACKED. Repeat in other direction
① THREAD THE NEEDLE straight leg means more rotation REPEAT 3 PER SIDE
Straighten one leg & tuck your toe under. Keep your hips level
Inhale: to lift arm & rotate
Exhale: to tuck arm & look under armpit
① TICK TOCK LEGS hip rotation with control REPEAT 4 PER SIDE
Press arms into floor. Legs squeezed together.
sink middle tummy
Exhale: rock legs to right & turn head to left. Use abdominals
Inhale to centre
Exhale: rock legs to left & turn head right
③ ROCKING RIBS strong rotation using the obliques REPEAT 4-8
Link hands behind head
Inhale: curl forward.
Exhale: rotate ribs to right
Inhale: centre
Exhale: rotate to left
*Make sure you turn cleanly on your axis
③ TORSO TWISTS stronger rotation with lifted legs REPEAT 4-8
Inhale: hold position
Exhale: twist torso one way & hips the other
Inhale: centre
Exhale: twist to the other side
THEN MAKE IT HARDER
Inhale: centre to deepen curl
Exhale: twist torso right, legs left, then straighten them
Inhale: bend knees & centre
Exhale: repeat other side

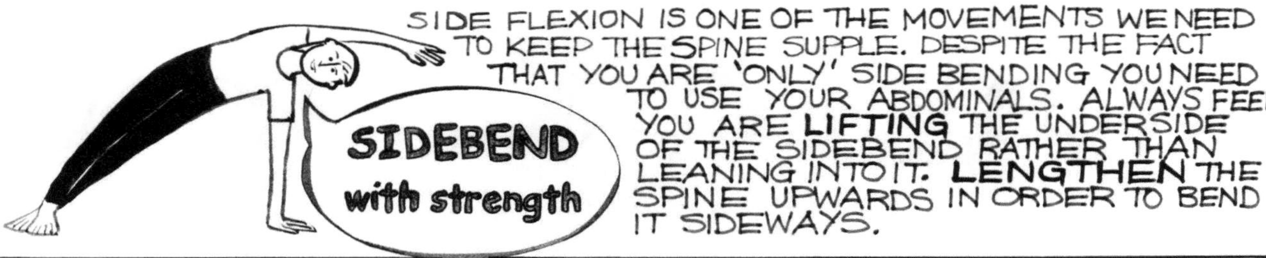

SIDE FLEXION IS ONE OF THE MOVEMENTS WE NEED TO KEEP THE SPINE SUPPLE. DESPITE THE FACT THAT YOU ARE 'ONLY' SIDE BENDING YOU NEED TO USE YOUR ABDOMINALS. ALWAYS FEEL YOU ARE **LIFTING** THE UNDERSIDE OF THE SIDEBEND RATHER THAN LEANING INTO IT. **LENGTHEN** THE SPINE UPWARDS IN ORDER TO BEND IT SIDEWAYS.

① STANDING SIDE BENDS — REPEAT 4 PER SIDE

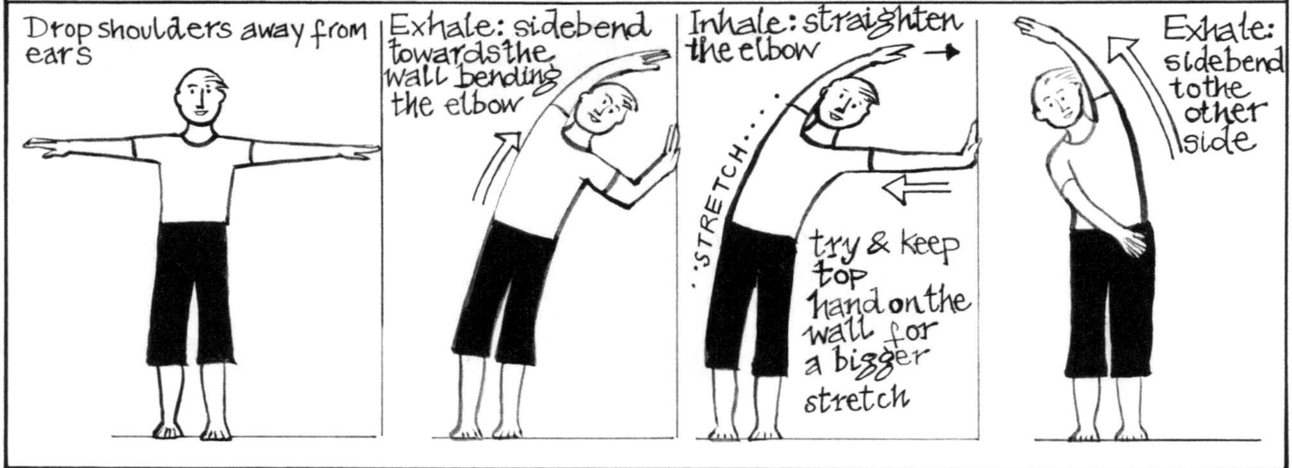

Drop shoulders away from ears

Exhale: sidebend towards the wall bending the elbow

Inhale: straighten the elbow →

STRETCH....

try & keep top hand on the wall for a bigger stretch

Exhale: sidebend to the other side

② MERMAID SIDE BENDS I — REPEAT 3 PER SIDE

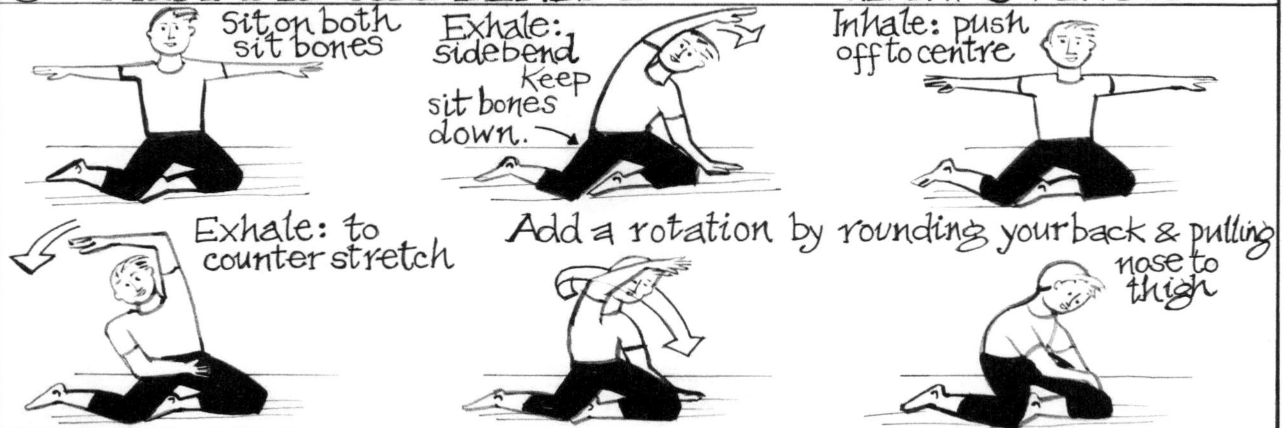

Sit on both sit bones

Exhale: sidebend

keep sit bones down.

Inhale: push off to centre

Exhale: to counter stretch

Add a rotation by rounding your back & pulling nose to thigh

③ MERMAID SIDEBENDS II — REPEAT 3 PER SIDE

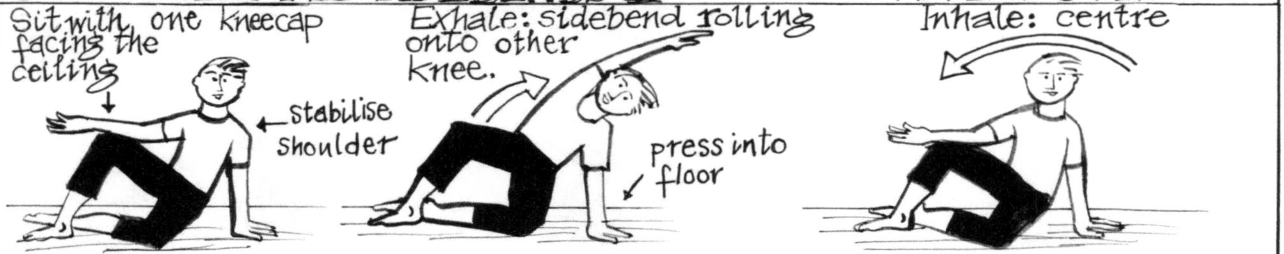

Sit with one kneecap facing the ceiling

← stabilise shoulder

Exhale: sidebend rolling onto other knee.

press into floor

Inhale: centre

④ BIG SIDEBENDS & TWISTS — REPEAT 3 PER SIDE

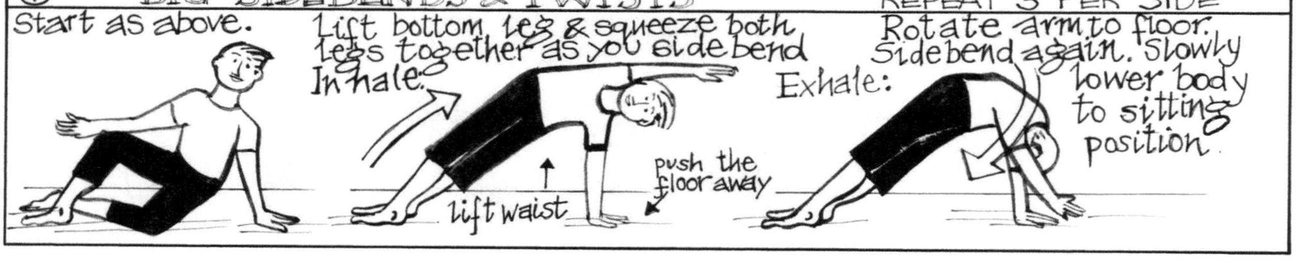

Start as above.

Lift bottom leg & squeeze both legs together as you sidebend

Inhale:

lift waist

push the floor away

Rotate arm to floor. Sidebend again.

Exhale:

Slowly lower body to sitting position

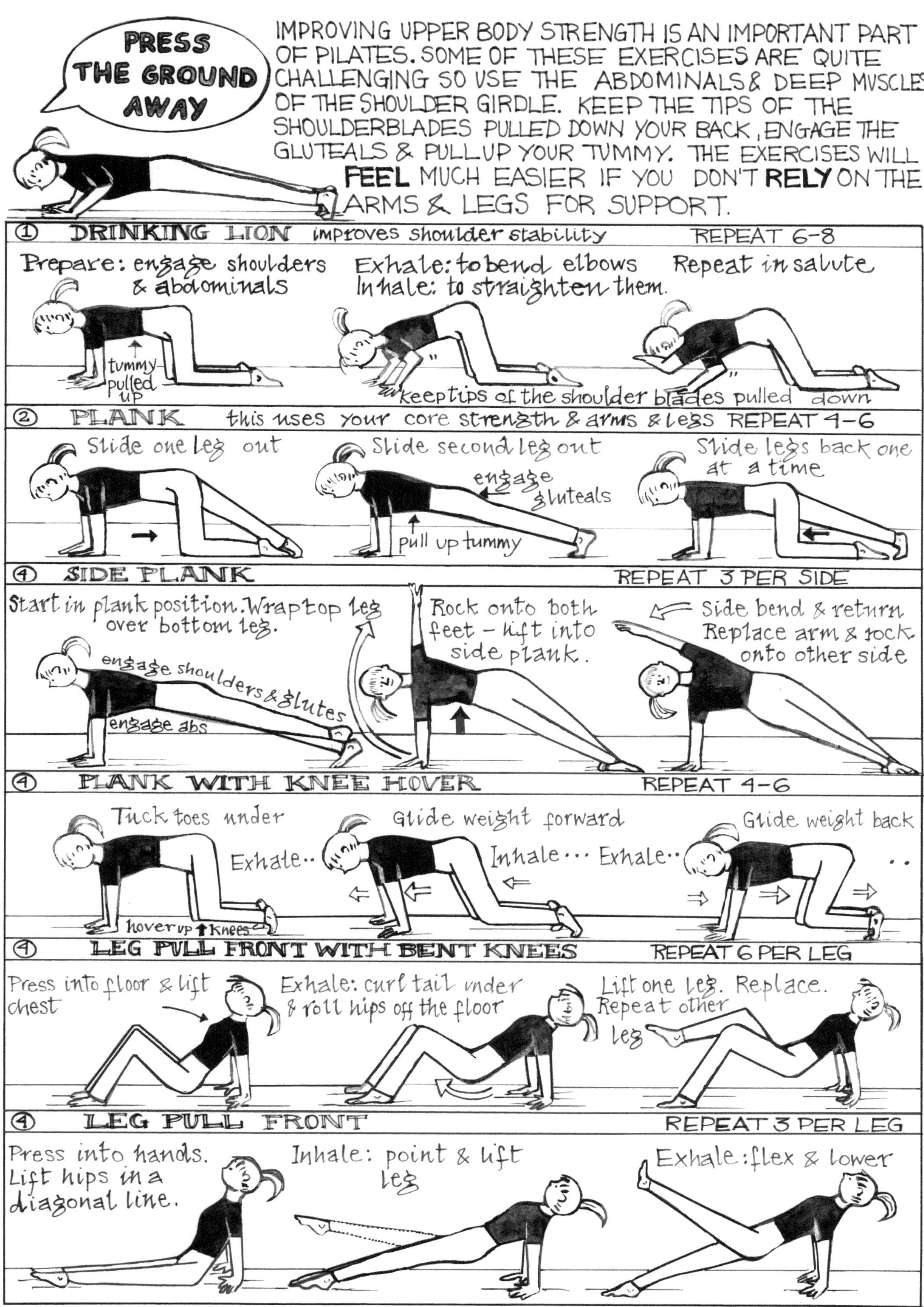
PRESS THE GROUND AWAY
IMPROVING UPPER BODY STRENGTH IS AN IMPORTANT PART OF PILATES. SOME OF THESE EXERCISES ARE QUITE CHALLENGING SO USE THE ABDOMINALS & DEEP MUSCLES OF THE SHOULDER GIRDLE. KEEP THE TIPS OF THE SHOULDERBLADES PULLED DOWN YOUR BACK, ENGAGE THE GLUTEALS & PULL UP YOUR TUMMY. THE EXERCISES WILL FEEL MUCH EASIER IF YOU DON'T RELY ON THE ARMS & LEGS FOR SUPPORT.
① DRINKING LION improves shoulder stability REPEAT 6-8
Prepare: engage shoulders & abdominals
Exhale: to bend elbows Inhale: to straighten them.
Repeat in salute
tummy pulled up
keep tips of the shoulder blades pulled down
② PLANK this uses your core strength & arms & legs REPEAT 4-6
Slide one leg out
Slide second leg out
engage gluteals
pull up tummy
Slide legs back one at a time
④ SIDE PLANK REPEAT 3 PER SIDE
Start in plank position. Wrap top leg over bottom leg.
engage shoulders & glutes
engage abs
Rock onto both feet – lift into side plank.
Side bend & return Replace arm & rock onto other side
④ PLANK WITH KNEE HOVER REPEAT 4-6
Tuck toes under
Exhale..
hover up knees
Glide weight forward
Inhale... Exhale..
Glide weight back
④ LEG PULL FRONT WITH BENT KNEES REPEAT 6 PER LEG
Press into floor & lift chest
Exhale: curl tail under & roll hips off the floor
Lift one leg. Replace. Repeat other leg
④ LEG PULL FRONT REPEAT 3 PER LEG
Press into hands. Lift hips in a diagonal line.
Inhale: point & lift leg
Exhale: flex & lower

Section 3

Pushing On

Try adding some of these higher level exercises to your workout. Be sensible and stop if anything hurts.

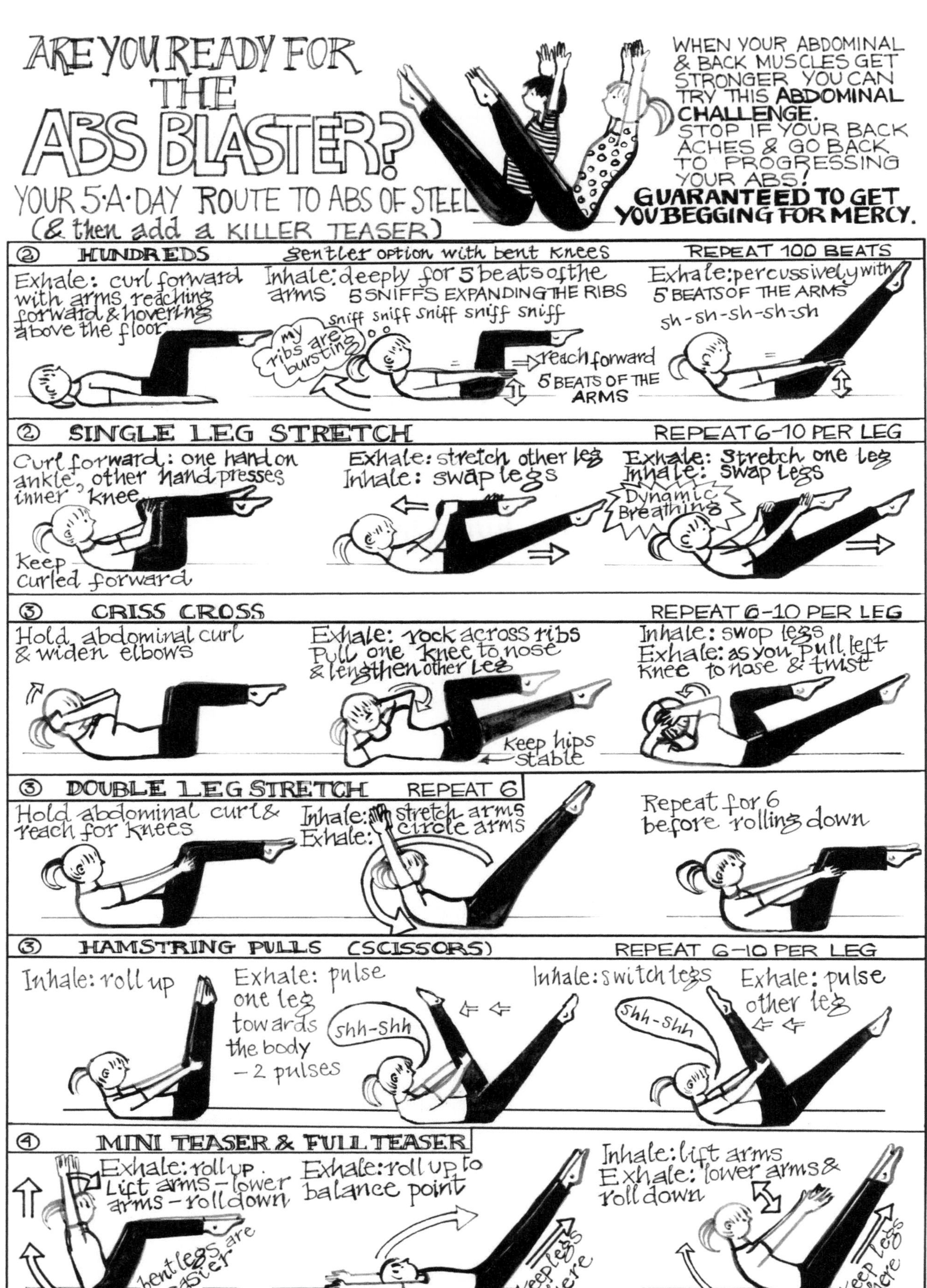
ARE YOU READY FOR THE ABS BLASTER?
YOUR 5·A·DAY ROUTE TO ABS OF STEEL
(& then add a KILLER TEASER)
WHEN YOUR ABDOMINAL & BACK MUSCLES GET STRONGER YOU CAN TRY THIS ABDOMINAL CHALLENGE. STOP IF YOUR BACK ACHES & GO BACK TO PROGRESSING YOUR ABS!
GUARANTEED TO GET YOU BEGGING FOR MERCY.
② HUNDREDS
gentler option with bent knees
REPEAT 100 BEATS
Exhale: curl forward with arms reaching forward & hovering above the floor
Inhale: deeply for 5 beats of the arms
5 SNIFFS EXPANDING THE RIBS
sniff sniff sniff sniff sniff
my ribs are bursting
reach forward
5 BEATS OF THE ARMS
Exhale: percussively with 5 BEATS OF THE ARMS
sh-sh-sh-sh-sh
② SINGLE LEG STRETCH
REPEAT 6-10 PER LEG
Curl forward: one hand on ankle, other hand presses inner knee
Keep curled forward
Exhale: stretch other leg
Inhale: swap legs
Exhale: Stretch one leg
Inhale: Swap Legs
Dynamic Breathing
③ CRISS CROSS
REPEAT 6-10 PER LEG
Hold abdominal curl & widen elbows
Exhale: rock across ribs
Pull one knee to nose & lengthen other leg
Keep hips stable
Inhale: swop legs
Exhale: as you pull left knee to nose & twist
③ DOUBLE LEG STRETCH
REPEAT 6
Hold abdominal curl & reach for knees
Inhale: stretch arms
Exhale: circle arms
Repeat for 6 before rolling down
③ HAMSTRING PULLS (SCISSORS)
REPEAT 6-10 PER LEG
Inhale: roll up
Exhale: pulse one leg towards the body – 2 pulses
shh-shh
Inhale: switch legs
Exhale: pulse other leg
Shh-Shh
④ MINI TEASER & FULL TEASER
Exhale: roll up. Lift arms – lower arms – roll down
bent legs are easier
Exhale: roll up to balance point
Keep legs here
Inhale: lift arms
Exhale: lower arms & roll down
Keep Legs here

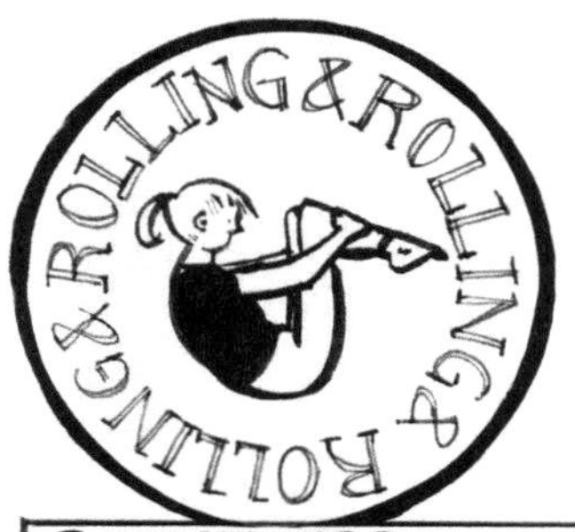

ROLLING LIKE A BALL IS A CLASSIC PILATES EXERCISE THAT DEMANDS STRONG ABDOMINALS & A FLEXIBLE LOW BACK. THIS SERIES OF EXERCISES IS DESIGNED TO INCREASE ABDOMINAL STRENGTH & FLEXIBILITY & HELP YOU ENJOY ROLLING & MASSAGING YOUR SPINAL MUSCLES. PERSISTING WITH YOUR ROLLING PRACTICE IS WORTH THE EFFORT AS THE EXERCISES STIMULATE THE SPINE & DEEPLY WORK THE ABDOMINAL MUSCLES. (AVOID IF YOU HAVE OSTEOPOROSIS, DISK ISSUES OR ARE PREGNANT)

② THE EGG — *imagine you have an egg balanced on your lap* — REPEAT 4

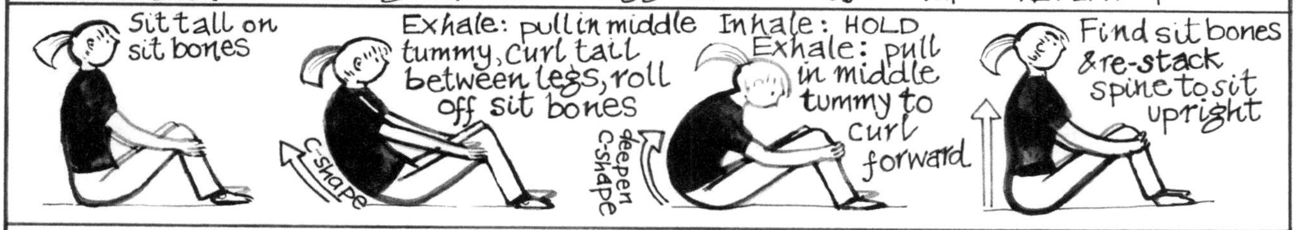

Sit tall on sit bones

Exhale: pull in middle tummy, curl tail between legs, roll off sit bones (C-shape)

Inhale: HOLD
Exhale: pull in middle tummy to curl forward (deepen C-shape)

Find sit bones & re-stack spine to sit upright

② EGG 2 — *lift the legs, balance but don't crush the egg* — REPEAT 4

Inhale: sit tall on sit bones

Exhale: curl tail between legs & roll off sit bones (pull in middle tummy)

Inhale: hold shape as you hover legs (C-shape, "hover")

Exhale: rock forward to sit

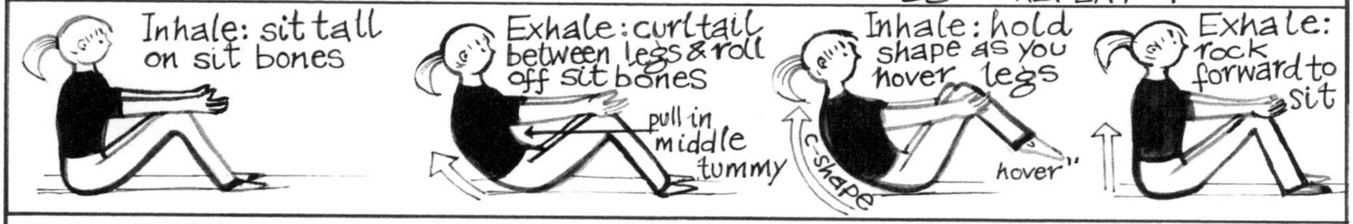

② EGG 3 — *lift legs, lift arms but don't crush the egg!* — REPEAT 4

Exhale: roll off sit bones

Hover legs
Deepen middle tummy (hover)

Inhale: lift arms (middle tummy, C-shape)

Rock Forward

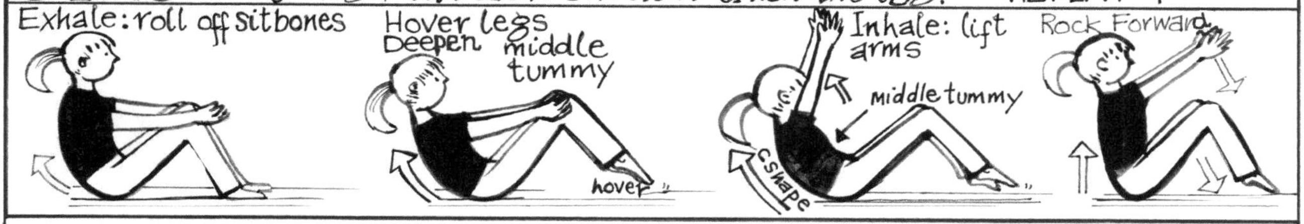

③ ABS-LEGS-ABS — *balance & change shape* — REPEAT 4

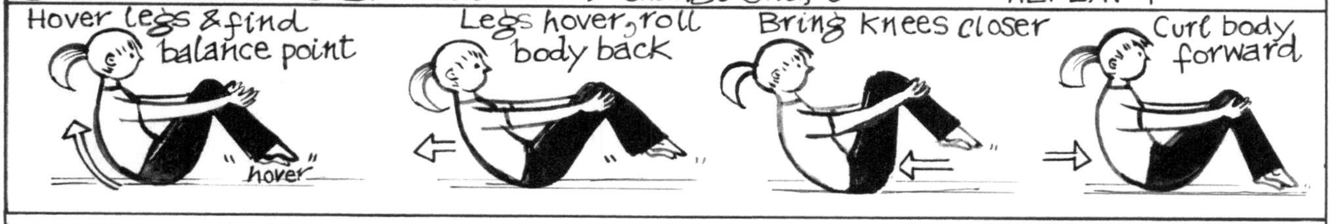

Hover legs & find balance point ("hover")

Legs hover, roll body back

Bring knees closer

Curl body forward

③ ROLL LIKE A BALL — *hold shape & roll* — REPEAT 4-6

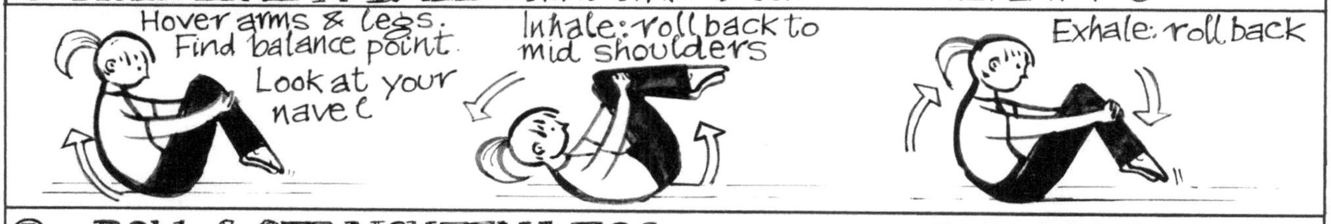

Hover arms & legs. Find balance point. Look at your navel

Inhale: roll back to mid shoulders

Exhale: roll back

③ ROLL & STRAIGHTEN LEGS — REPEAT 4-6

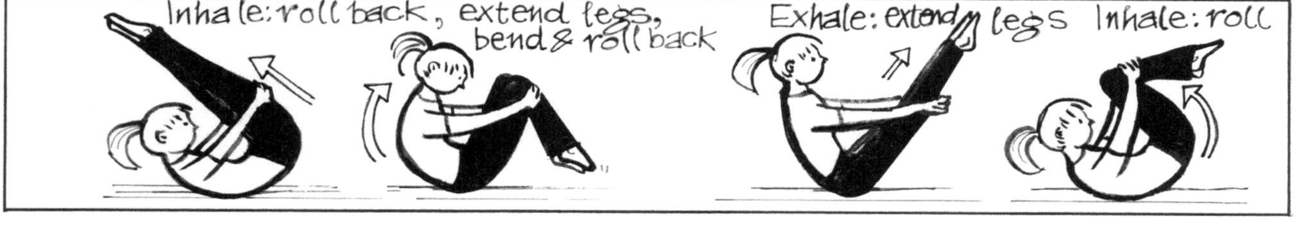

Inhale: roll back, extend legs, bend & roll back

Exhale: extend legs

Inhale: roll

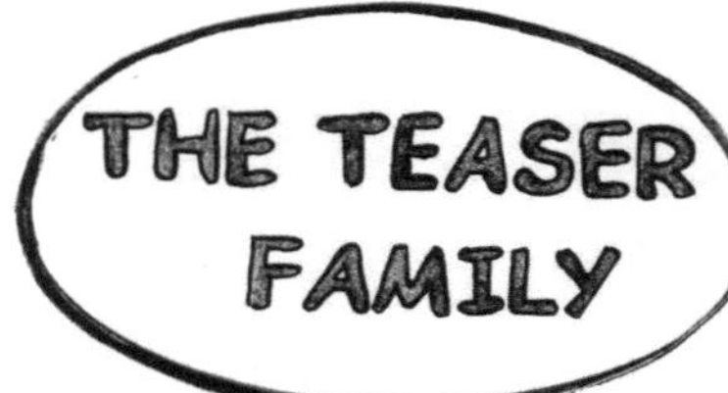

THESE ABDOMINAL EXERCISES ARE SOME OF THE MOST DAUNTING IN THE PILATES REPERTOIRE & FORCE YOU TO USE YOUR DEEP ABDOMINAL MUSCLES. YOU CANNOT CHEAT & JUST USE YOUR HIP FLEXORS. WHY ARE THEY CALLED TEASERS? NO ONE KNOWS, BUT THEY REQUIRE BALANCE, STRENGTH & A SENSE OF HUMOUR.

START WITH NO1 BUT ONLY MOVE ON WHEN YOU'VE MASTERED IT.

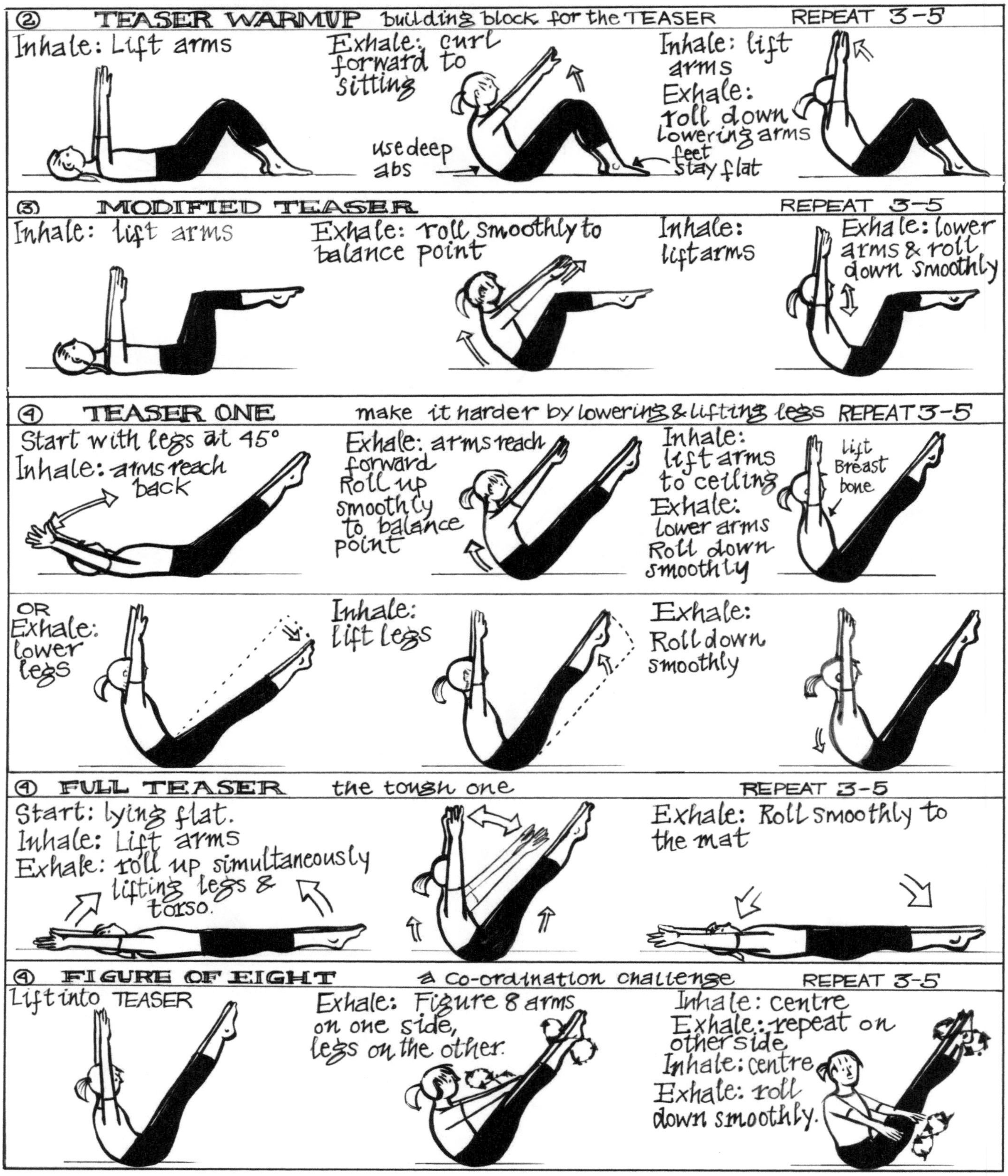

② TEASER WARMUP — building block for the TEASER — REPEAT 3-5

Inhale: Lift arms

Exhale: curl forward to sitting (use deep abs)

Inhale: lift arms
Exhale: roll down lowering arms (feet stay flat)

③ MODIFIED TEASER — REPEAT 3-5

Inhale: lift arms

Exhale: roll smoothly to balance point

Inhale: lift arms

Exhale: lower arms & roll down smoothly

④ TEASER ONE — make it harder by lowering & lifting legs — REPEAT 3-5

Start with legs at 45°
Inhale: arms reach back

Exhale: arms reach forward
Roll up smoothly to balance point

Inhale: lift arms to ceiling (lift Breast bone)
Exhale: lower arms
Roll down smoothly

OR
Exhale: lower legs

Inhale: lift legs

Exhale: Roll down smoothly

④ FULL TEASER — the tough one — REPEAT 3-5

Start: lying flat.
Inhale: Lift arms
Exhale: roll up simultaneously lifting legs & torso.

Exhale: Roll smoothly to the mat

④ FIGURE OF EIGHT — a co-ordination challenge — REPEAT 3-5

Lift into TEASER

Exhale: Figure 8 arms on one side, legs on the other.

Inhale: centre
Exhale: repeat on other side
Inhale: centre
Exhale: roll down smoothly.

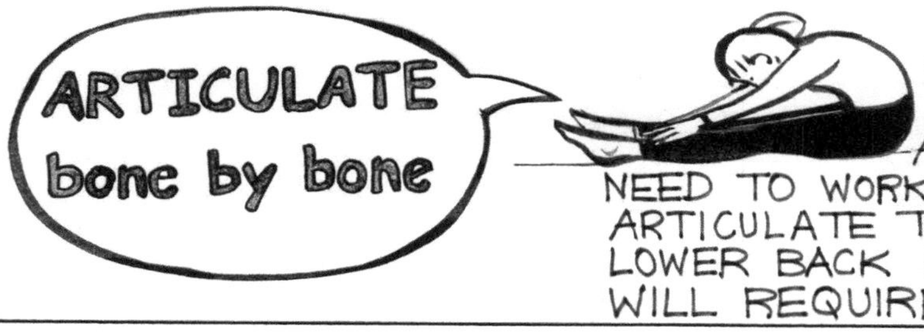

ARTICULATE bone by bone

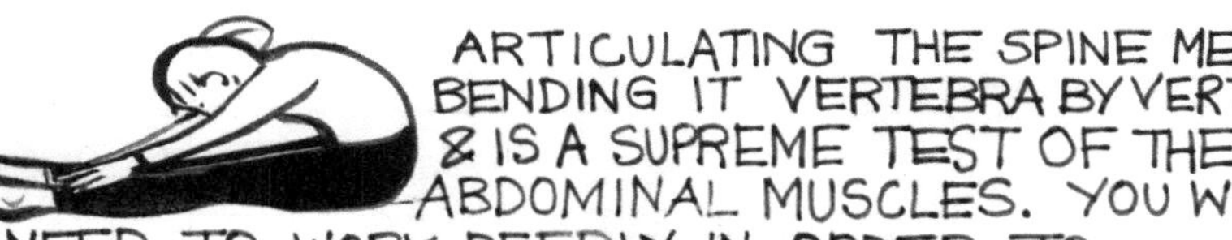

ARTICULATING THE SPINE MEANS BENDING IT VERTEBRA BY VERTEBRA & IS A SUPREME TEST OF THE ABDOMINAL MUSCLES. YOU WILL NEED TO WORK DEEPLY IN ORDER TO ARTICULATE THE LUMBAR SPINE & IF THE LOWER BACK IS STIFF THESE EXERCISES WILL REQUIRE SOME PRACTICE.

② ROLL BACK — warm up your abdominals & back — REPEAT 4–6

Inhale: sit up tall

Exhale: hollow middle tummy. Create a "C" curve & roll back

"C" curve

eventually roll to the floor

Inhale: hold position
Exhale: roll forward

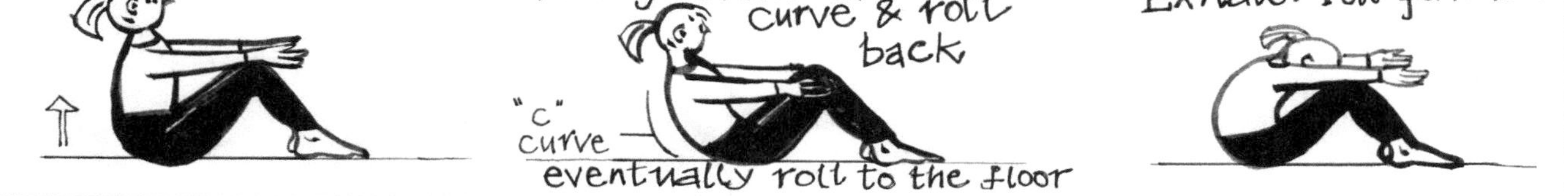

② SPINE STRETCH — a mid back stretch — REPEAT 4–6

Sit upright
Legs in a narrow "V" shape

Exhale: scoop middle tummy to round the spine
Inhale: roll upright

pull in here

"C" curve

If hamstrings are tight bend the knees

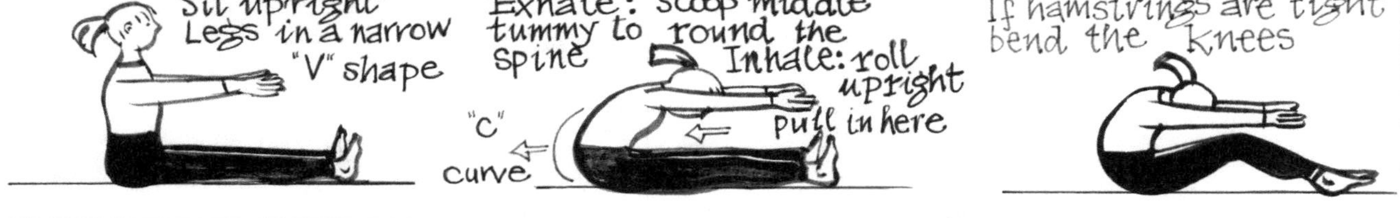

③ ROLL UP — Try this when you've mastered ROLL BACK — REPEAT 4–6

Inhale: stretch out & squeeze legs together

Exhale: lift arms ..

Roll up-arms in line with shoulders

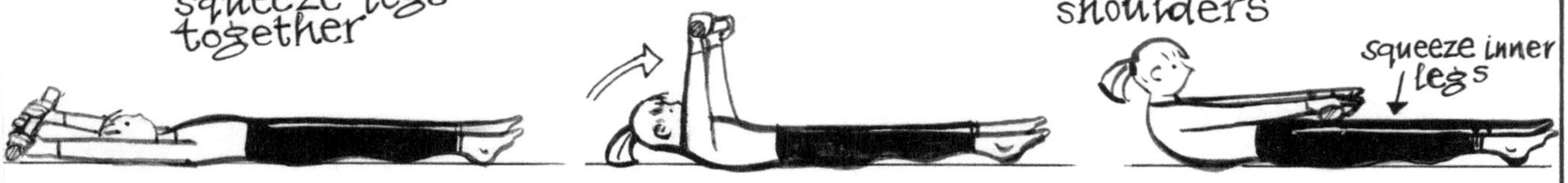

squeeze inner legs

Inhale: lean forward

keep "C" curve

use abs

Exhale: roll back one • bone • at • a • time ...

Inhale: stretch out & repeat

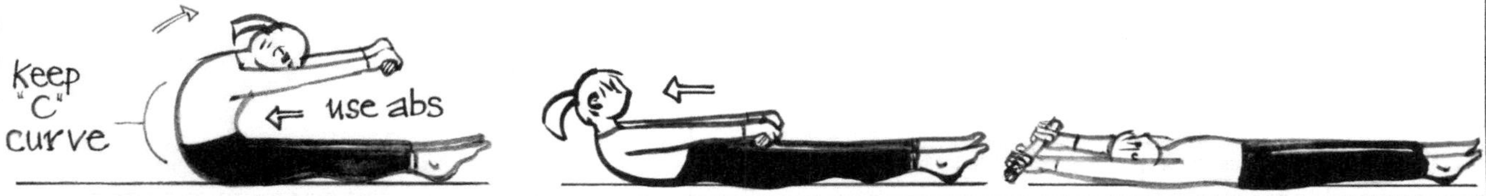

④ NECK PULL — a super tough roll up (DO NOT PULL THE NECK) REPEAT 4

Inhale: flex feet, dig heels into the mat

legs in a narrow "V" shape

Exhale: roll up.
Use gluteals
Press legs into the mat

Continue to roll forwards

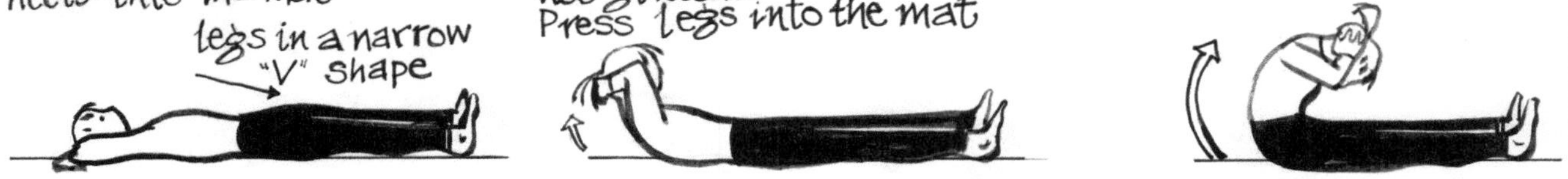

Inhale: Stack the spine

Exhale: roll back one bone at a time

scoop abdominals

create "C" curve

Roll to the mat with control.

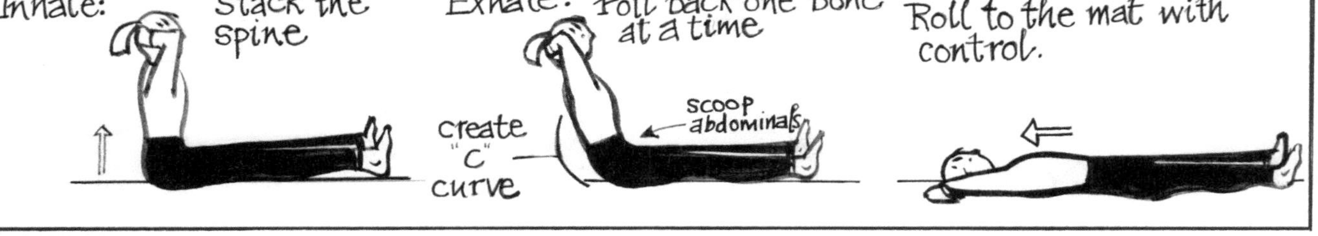

GO UPSIDE DOWN

The Inverted postures

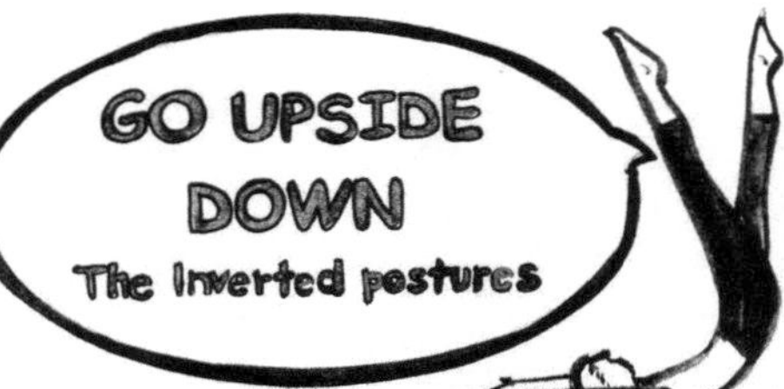

OK, SO THINGS ARE GETTING MORE DIFFICULT & YOU NEED PLENTY OF "CORE" STRENGTH FOR THESE. THEY TEACH SPINAL ARTICULATION & BALANCE. IF YOU HAVE PROBLEMS GETTING YOUR HIPS UP, HAVE A TIGHT BACK OR HAMSTRINGS CONTINUE TO PRACTICE THE 'HIP UP PRACTICE' BELOW.

Inverted postures are unsuitable if you have neck problems, osteoporosis, high blood pressure or are pregnant.

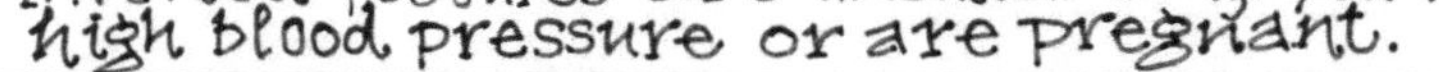

④ ROLLOVER — REPEAT 6-8

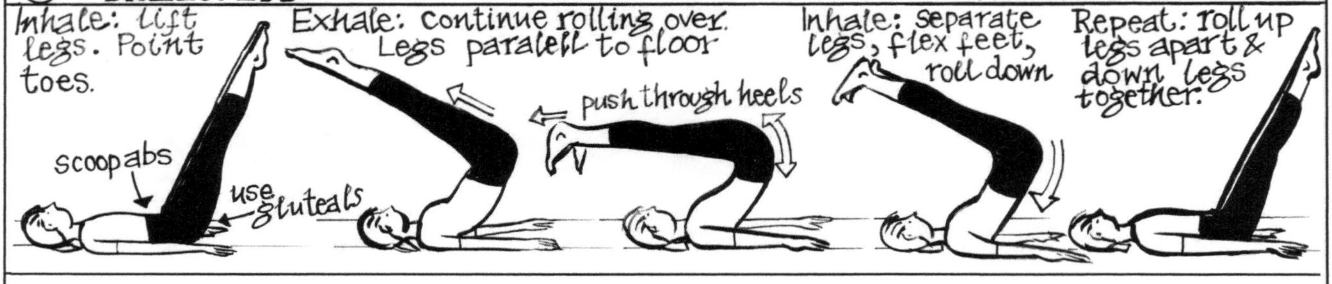

Inhale: lift legs. Point toes.
scoop abs
use gluteals
Exhale: continue rolling over. Legs paralell to floor
push through heels
Inhale: separate legs, flex feet, roll down
Repeat: roll up legs apart & down legs together.

④ JACKKNIFE — A dynamic rollover demanding strong abs. REPEAT 3

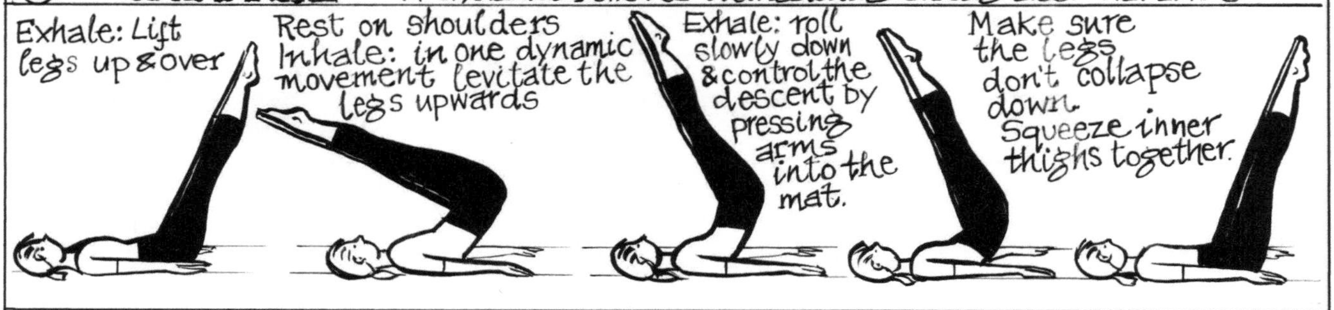

Exhale: Lift legs up & over
Rest on shoulders
Inhale: in one dynamic movement levitate the legs upwards
Exhale: roll slowly down & control the descent by pressing arms into the mat.
Make sure the legs don't collapse down.
Squeeze inner thighs together.

④ OPEN LEG ROCKER — harder than roll like a ball — REPEAT 4-6

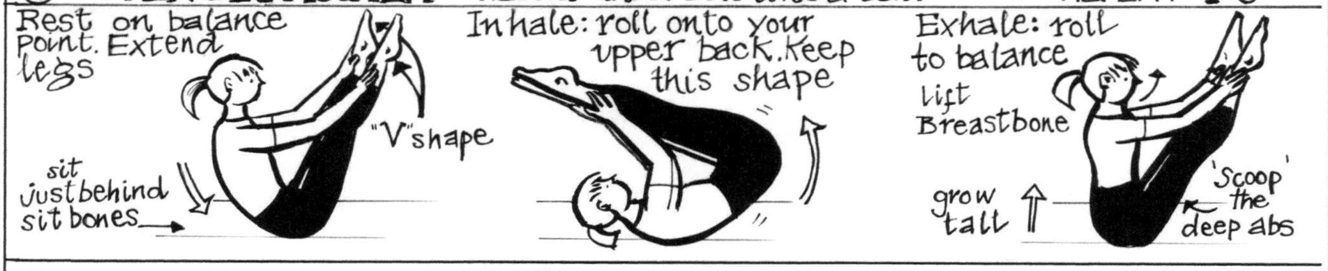

Rest on balance point. Extend legs
"V" shape
sit just behind sit bones
Inhale: roll onto your upper back. Keep this shape
Exhale: roll to balance
lift Breastbone
grow tall
'Scoop' the deep abs

④ CONTROL BALANCE — REPEAT 3-5 per leg

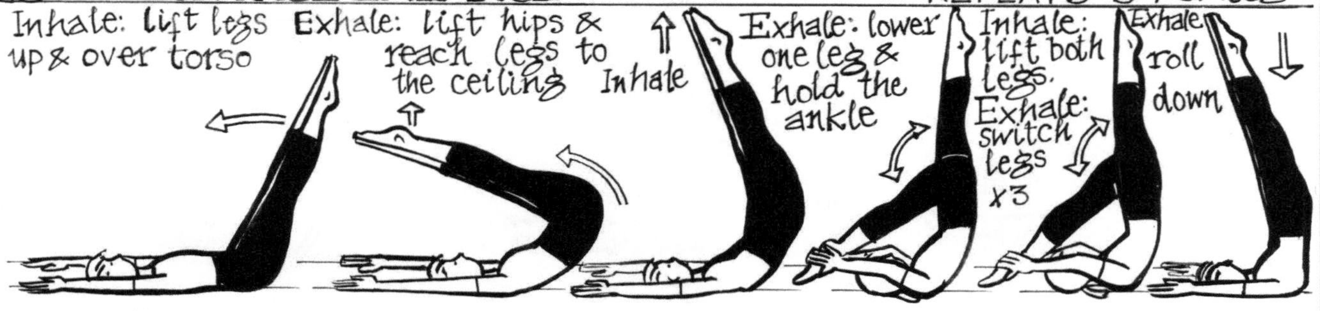

Inhale: lift legs up & over torso
Exhale: lift hips & reach legs to the ceiling
Inhale
Exhale: lower one leg & hold the ankle
Inhale: lift both legs.
Exhale: switch legs x3
Exhale roll down

HIP UP PRACTICE

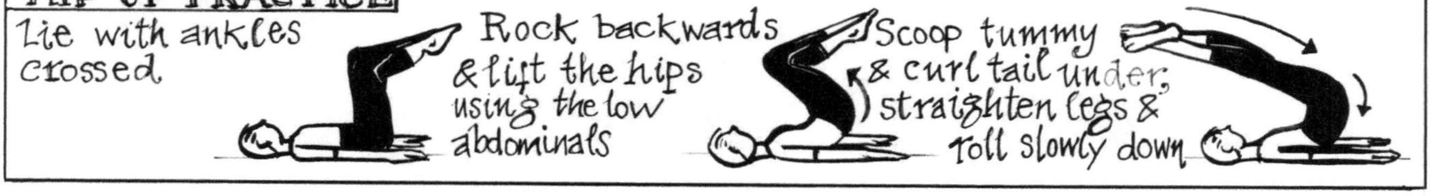

Lie with ankles crossed
Rock backwards & lift the hips using the low abdominals
Scoop tummy & curl tail under, straighten legs & roll slowly down

LEG CIRCLES
single & double

CIRCLING YOUR LEG MIGHT SEEM SIMPLE BUT KEEPING YOUR TORSO STABLE AT THE SAME TIME WITHOUT TENSION IS HARDER. PRACTICE NO1 & 2 TO GET THE ABDOMINALS WORKING & TO MOBILISE THE HIPS BEFORE YOU MOVE ONTO NO3. BE AWARE THAT DOUBLE LEG CIRCLES DEMAND STRENGTH & CONTROL.

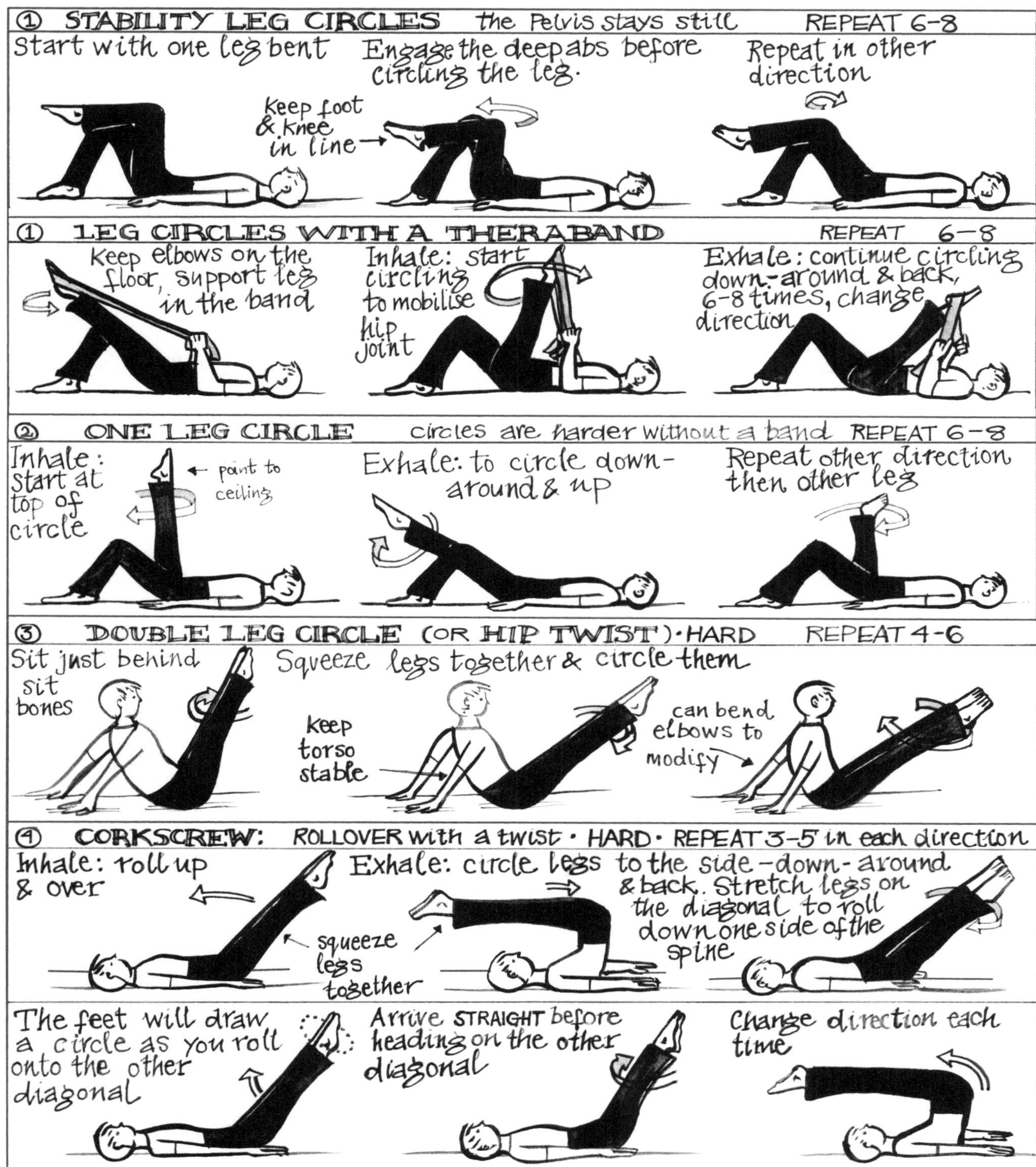

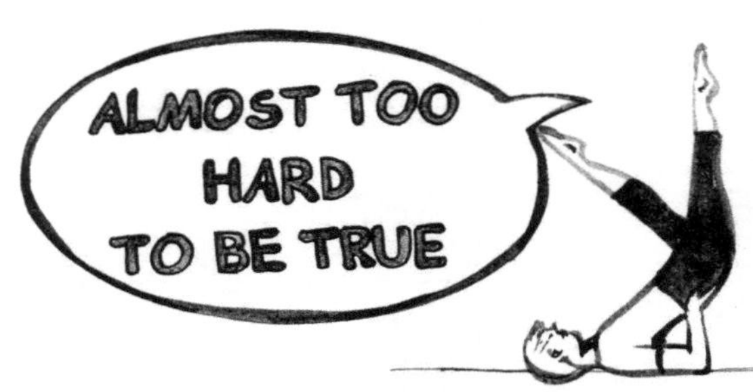

ALL THESE EXERCISES ARE PART OF THE ORIGINAL PILATES REPERTOIRE & ARE VERY 'STRONG' (PILATES SPEAK FOR REALLY REALLY HARD) SOME ARE EXERCISES YOU HAVE ALREADY TACKLED BUT WITH AN EXTRA ELEMENT OF BALANCE & CONTROL ADDED. THEY ARE ALL PART OF JO PILATES ORIGINAL 'CLASSICAL' REPERTOIRE.

④ SIDE KICK KNEELING — REPEAT 8–10

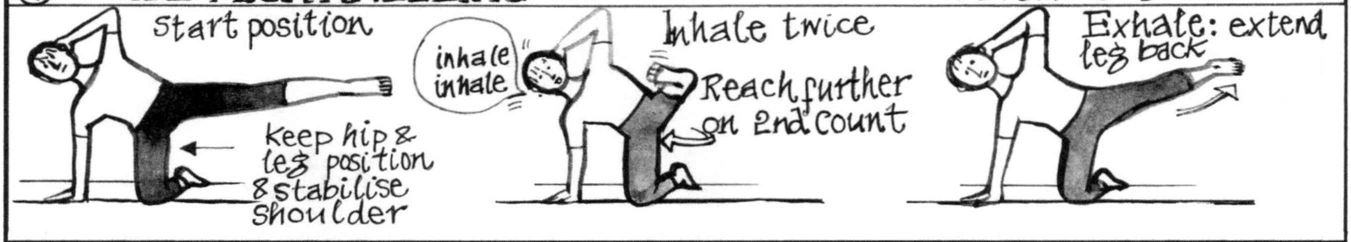

Start position. Keep hip & leg position & stabilise shoulder

Inhale twice (inhale inhale). Reach further on 2nd count

Exhale: extend leg back

④ SCISSORS IN THE AIR — REPEAT 5–10 SCISSORS

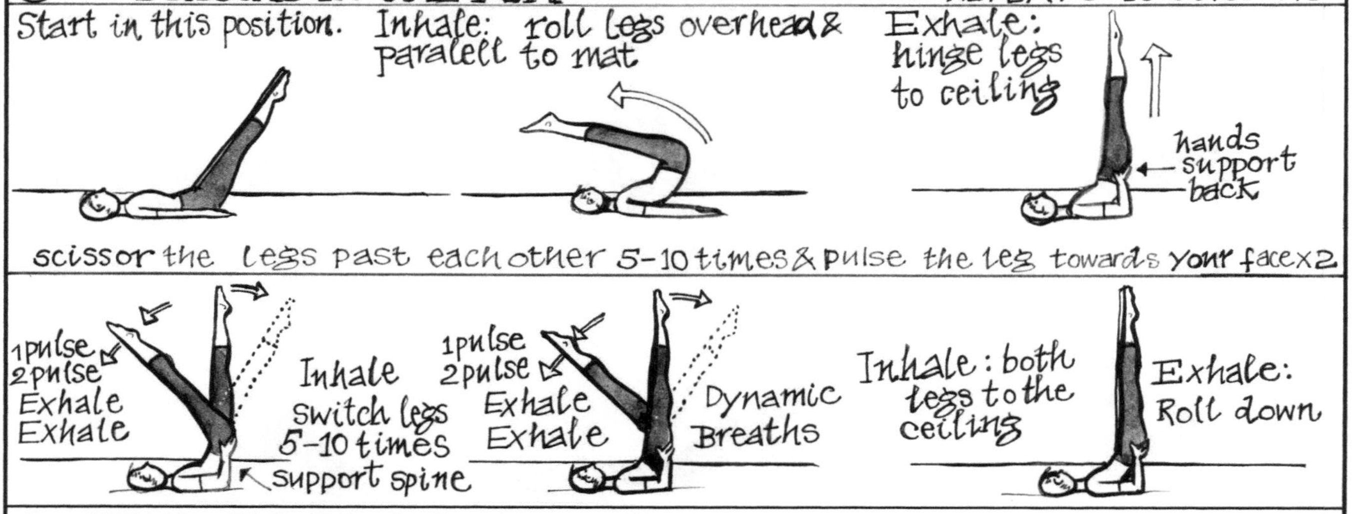

Start in this position.

Inhale: roll legs overhead & paralell to mat

Exhale: hinge legs to ceiling. Hands support back

scissor the legs past each other 5–10 times & pulse the leg towards your face x2

1 pulse 2 pulse Exhale Exhale. Inhale switch legs 5–10 times. Support spine

1 pulse 2 pulse Exhale Exhale. Dynamic Breaths

Inhale: both legs to the ceiling

Exhale: Roll down

④ BICYCLES IN THE AIR — REPEAT 5–10 BICYCLES, 5–10 IN REVERSE

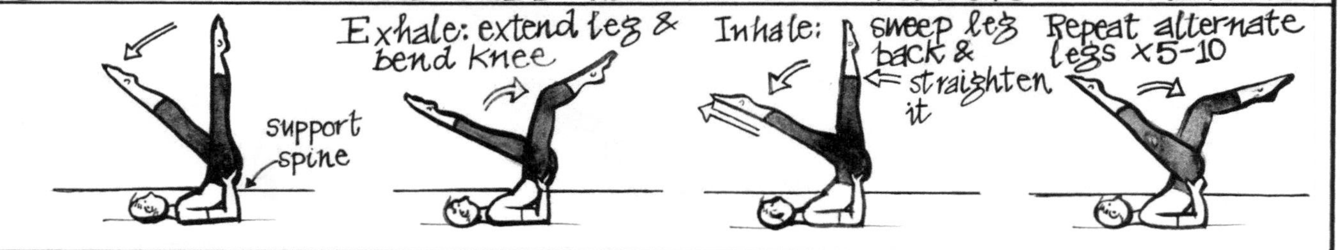

Support spine

Exhale: extend leg & bend knee

Inhale: sweep leg back & straighten it

Repeat alternate legs x5–10

④ THE SEAL (this makes everyone giggle!) — REPEAT 8–10

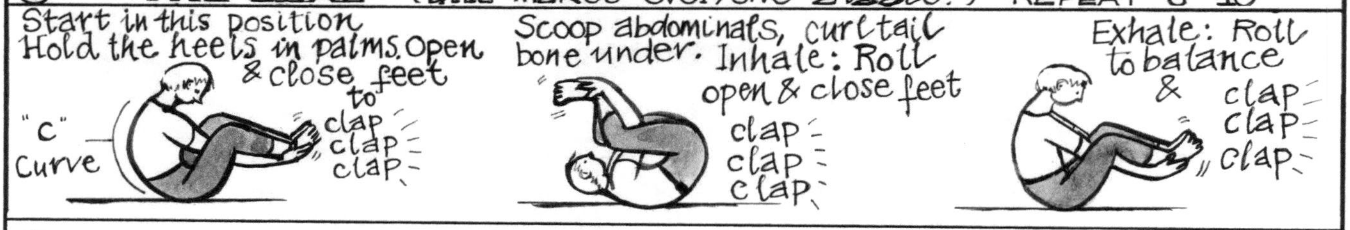

Start in this position. Hold the heels in palms. Open & close feet to clap clap clap. "C" Curve

Scoop abdominals, curl tail bone under. Inhale: Roll open & close feet clap clap clap

Exhale: Roll to balance & clap clap clap

⑤ CRAB — If you think the SEAL is weird, this is insane. BE CAREFUL!

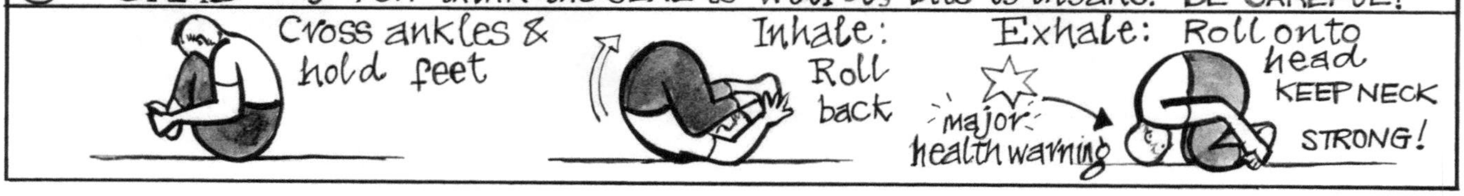

Cross ankles & hold feet

Inhale: Roll back

Exhale: Roll onto head. KEEP NECK STRONG! major health warning

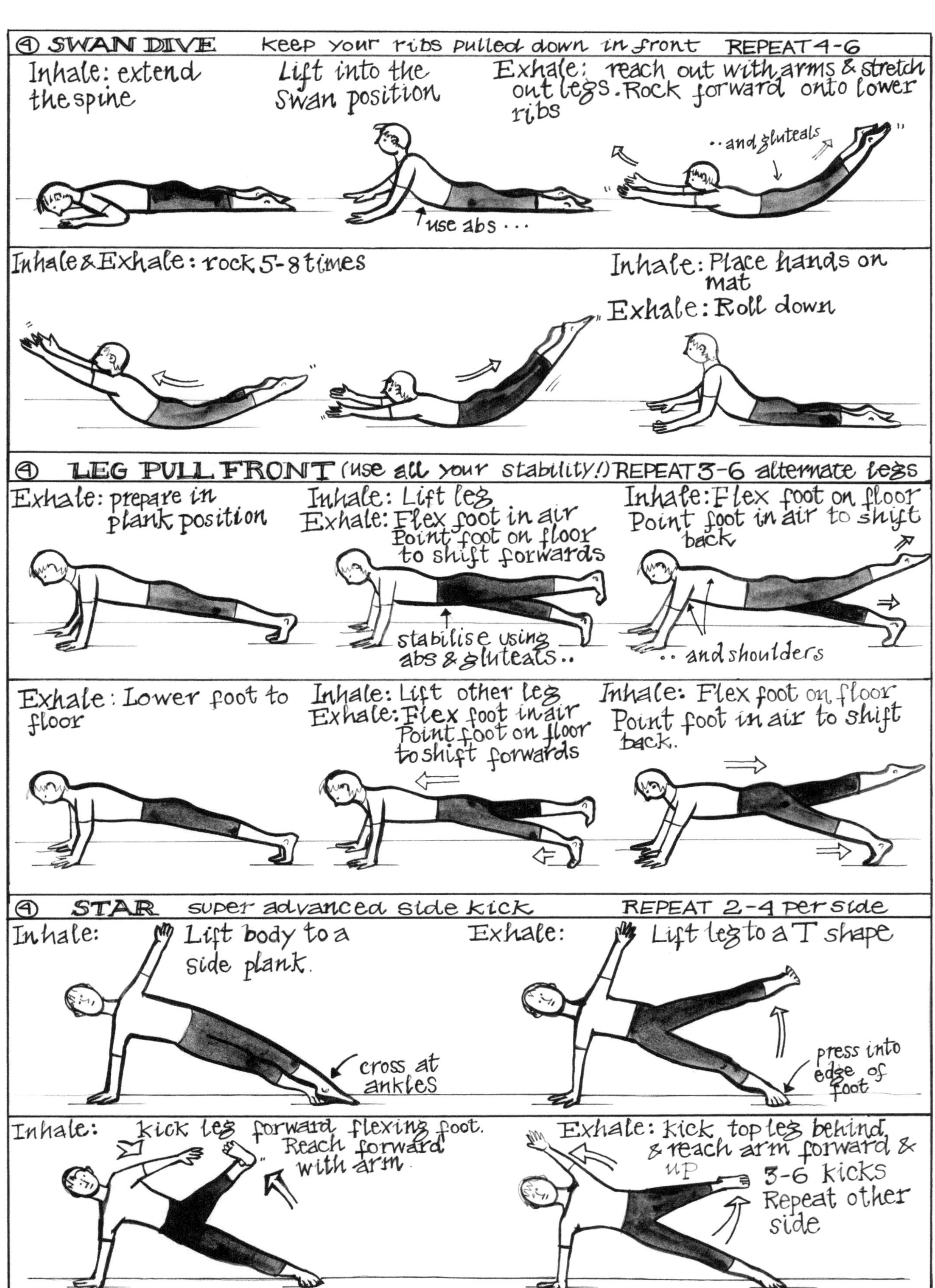

④ SWAN DIVE keep your ribs pulled down in front REPEAT 4-6
Inhale: extend the spine
Lift into the Swan position
Exhale: reach out with arms & stretch out legs. Rock forward onto lower ribs
..and gluteals
use abs...
Inhale & Exhale: rock 5-8 times
Inhale: Place hands on mat
Exhale: Roll down
④ LEG PULL FRONT (use all your stability!) REPEAT 3-6 alternate legs
Exhale: prepare in plank position
Inhale: Lift leg
Exhale: Flex foot in air
Point foot on floor to shift forwards
stabilise using abs & gluteals..
Inhale: Flex foot on floor
Point foot in air to shift back
.. and shoulders
Exhale: Lower foot to floor
Inhale: Lift other leg
Exhale: Flex foot in air
Point foot on floor to shift forwards
Inhale: Flex foot on floor
Point foot in air to shift back.
④ STAR super advanced side kick REPEAT 2-4 per side
Inhale: Lift body to a side plank.
cross at ankles
Exhale: Lift leg to a T shape
press into edge of foot
Inhale: kick leg forward flexing foot. Reach forward with arm.
Exhale: kick top leg behind & reach arm forward & up
3-6 kicks
Repeat other side

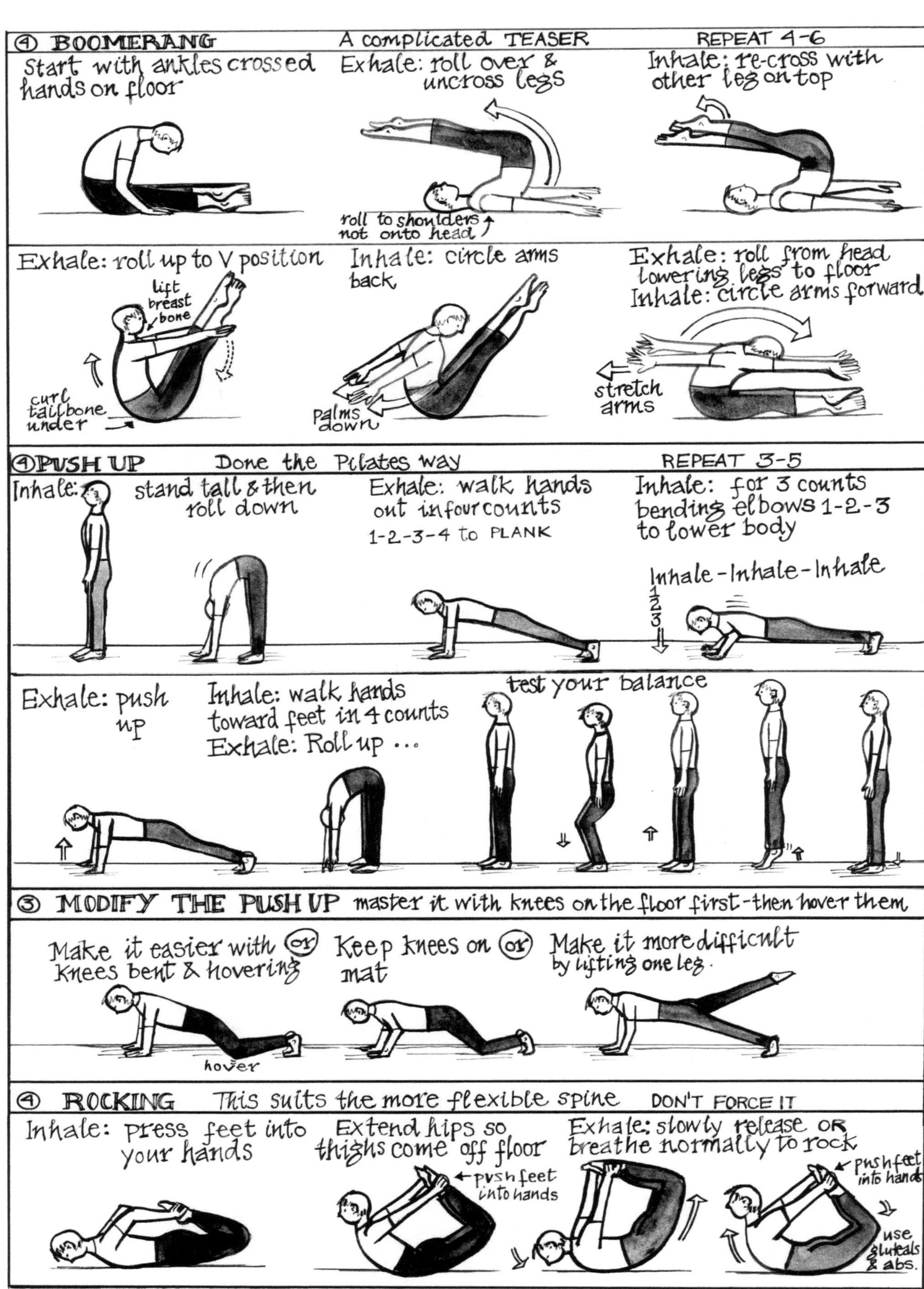

4 BOOMERANG
A complicated TEASER
REPEAT 4-6
Start with ankles crossed hands on floor
Exhale: roll over & uncross legs
Inhale: re-cross with other leg on top
roll to shoulders not onto head
Exhale: roll up to V position
lift breast bone
curl tailbone under
Inhale: circle arms back
palms down
Exhale: roll from head lowering legs to floor
Inhale: circle arms forward
stretch arms
4 PUSH UP
Done the Pilates way
REPEAT 3-5
Inhale: stand tall & then roll down
Exhale: walk hands out in four counts 1-2-3-4 to PLANK
Inhale: for 3 counts bending elbows 1-2-3 to lower body
Inhale-Inhale-Inhale
1
2
3
Exhale: push up
Inhale: walk hands toward feet in 4 counts
Exhale: Roll up ...
test your balance
3 MODIFY THE PUSH UP
master it with knees on the floor first-then hover them
Make it easier with knees bent & hovering
or
Keep knees on mat
or
Make it more difficult by lifting one leg.
hover
4 ROCKING
This suits the more flexible spine
DON'T FORCE IT
Inhale: press feet into your hands
Extend hips so thighs come off floor
push feet into hands
Exhale: slowly release or breathe normally to rock
push feet into hands
use gluteals & abs.

Section 4

A Workout a Day

In this section you will be introduced to a workout designed to flow from beginning to end. Over the years I have been lucky enough to take classes with many inspiring teachers some of whom have agreed to design a class for this book. Practice the exercises individually and then follow the class from beginning to end. Take your time and enjoy the movements.

Lyn's Daily Wake Up

YOU'VE SEEN YOUR DOG & CAT DO IT! KNEEL DOWN & ROUND YOUR BACK, LIE DOWN TO ROLL INTO A BRIDGE, ROLL YOUR HIPS FROM SIDE TO SIDE. LIE ON YOUR FRONT TO ARCH YOUR BACK.

FIND YOUR INNER ANIMAL

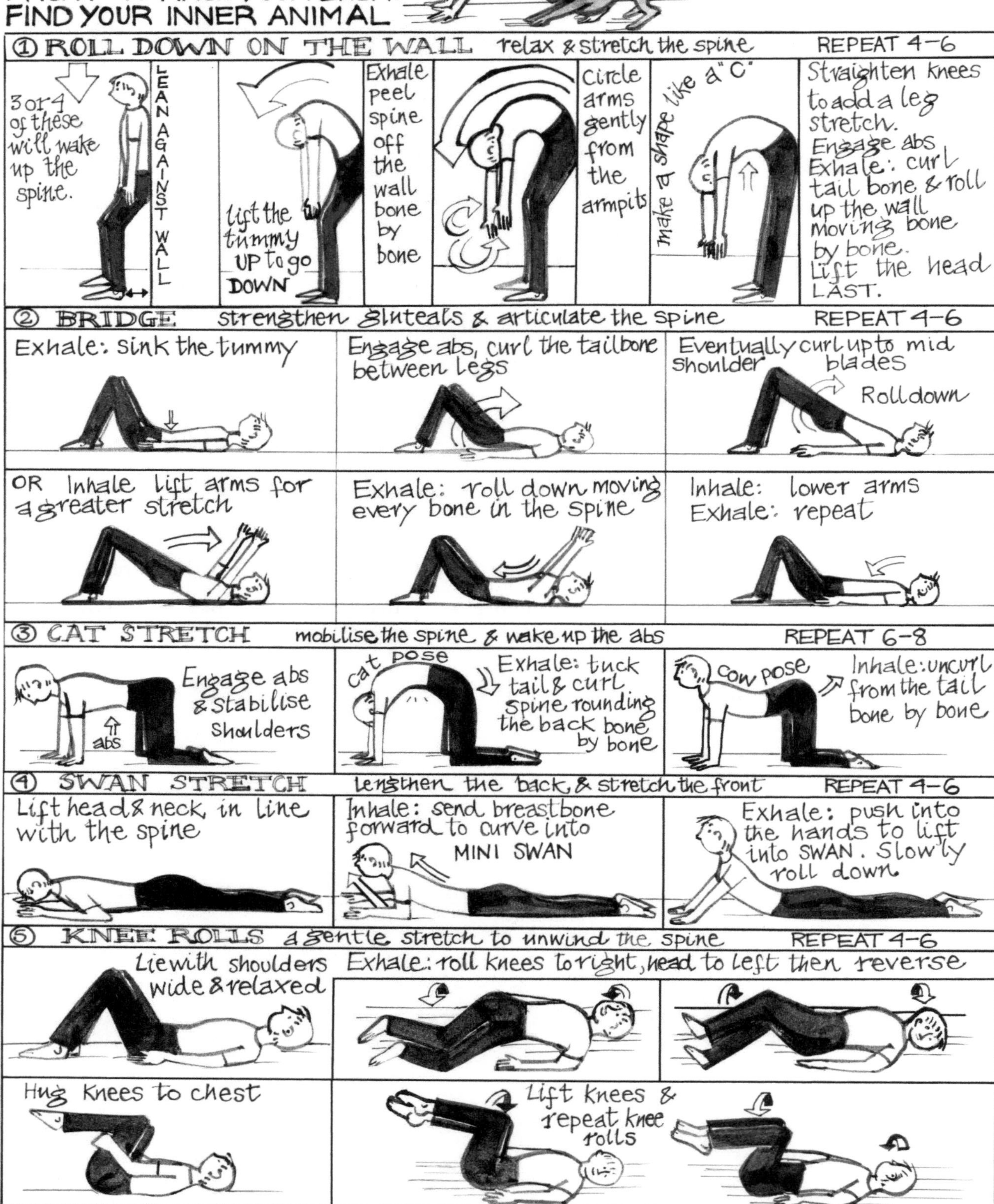

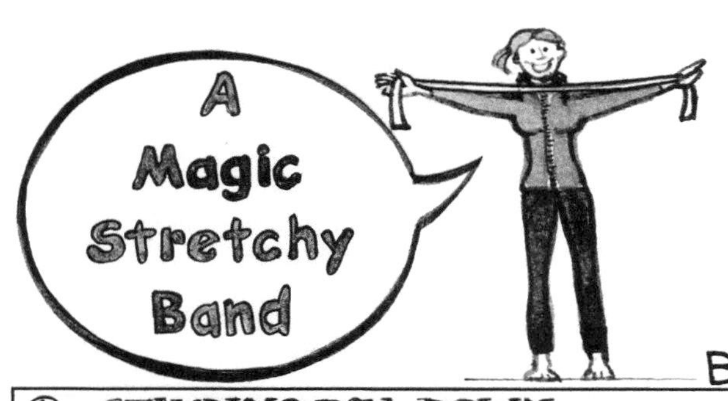

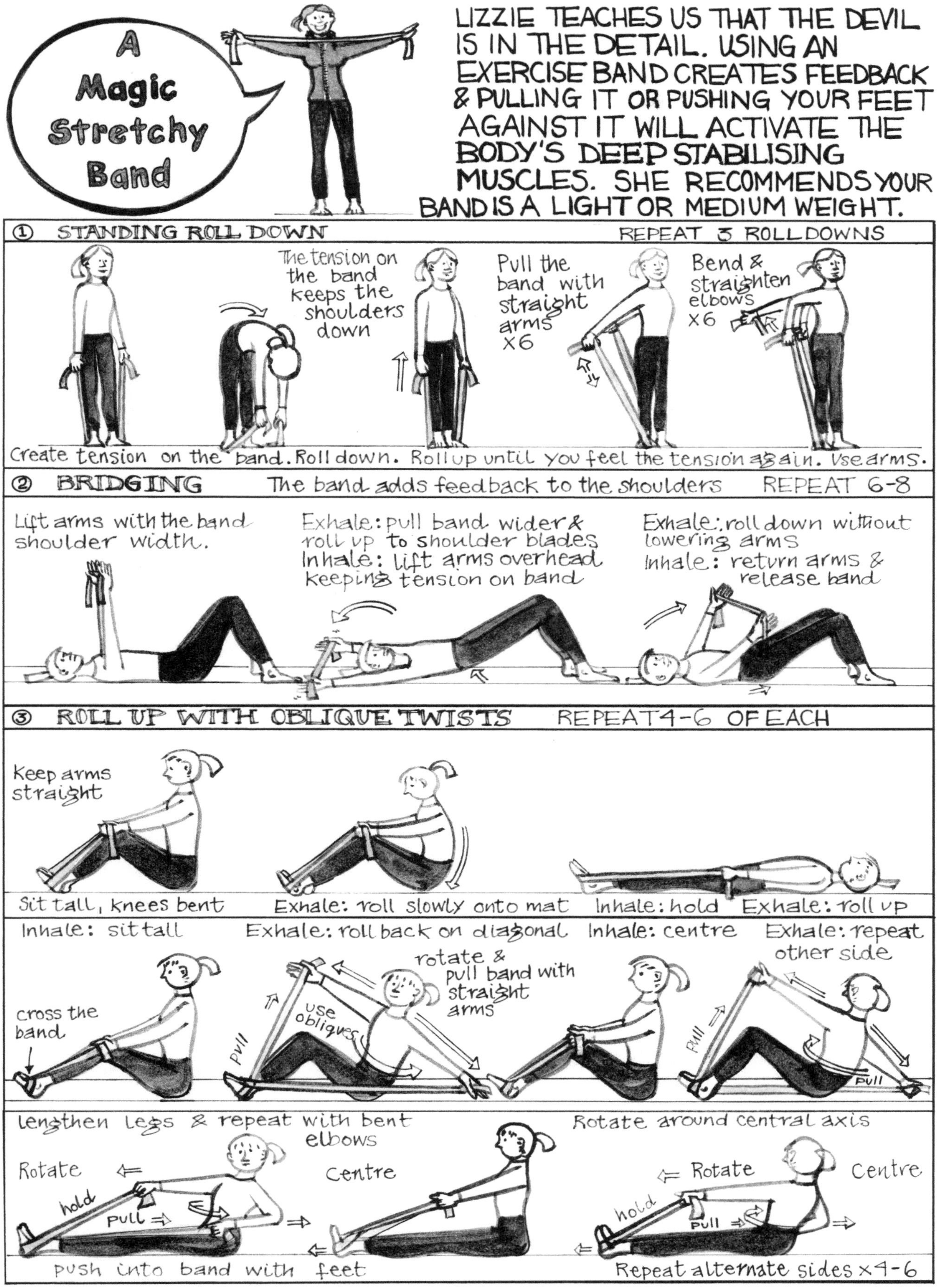

LIZZIE TEACHES US THAT THE DEVIL IS IN THE DETAIL. USING AN EXERCISE BAND CREATES FEEDBACK & PULLING IT OR PUSHING YOUR FEET AGAINST IT WILL ACTIVATE THE BODY'S DEEP STABILISING MUSCLES. SHE RECOMMENDS YOUR BAND IS A LIGHT OR MEDIUM WEIGHT.

① STANDING ROLL DOWN

REPEAT 3 ROLLDOWNS

The tension on the band keeps the shoulders down

Pull the band with straight arms X6

Bend & straighten elbows X6

Create tension on the band. Roll down. Roll up until you feel the tension again. Use arms.

② BRIDGING

The band adds feedback to the shoulders REPEAT 6-8

Lift arms with the band shoulder width.

Exhale: pull band wider & roll up to shoulder blades
Inhale: lift arms overhead keeping tension on band

Exhale: roll down without lowering arms
Inhale: return arms & release band

③ ROLL UP WITH OBLIQUE TWISTS

REPEAT 4-6 OF EACH

Keep arms straight

Sit tall, knees bent

Exhale: roll slowly onto mat

Inhale: hold Exhale: roll up

Inhale: sit tall

cross the band

Exhale: roll back on diagonal

rotate & pull band with straight arms

use obliques

pull

Inhale: centre

Exhale: repeat other side

pull

pull

lengthen legs & repeat with bent elbows

Rotate

hold

pull

Centre

push into band with feet

Rotate around central axis

Rotate

Centre

hold

pull

Repeat alternate sides x4-6

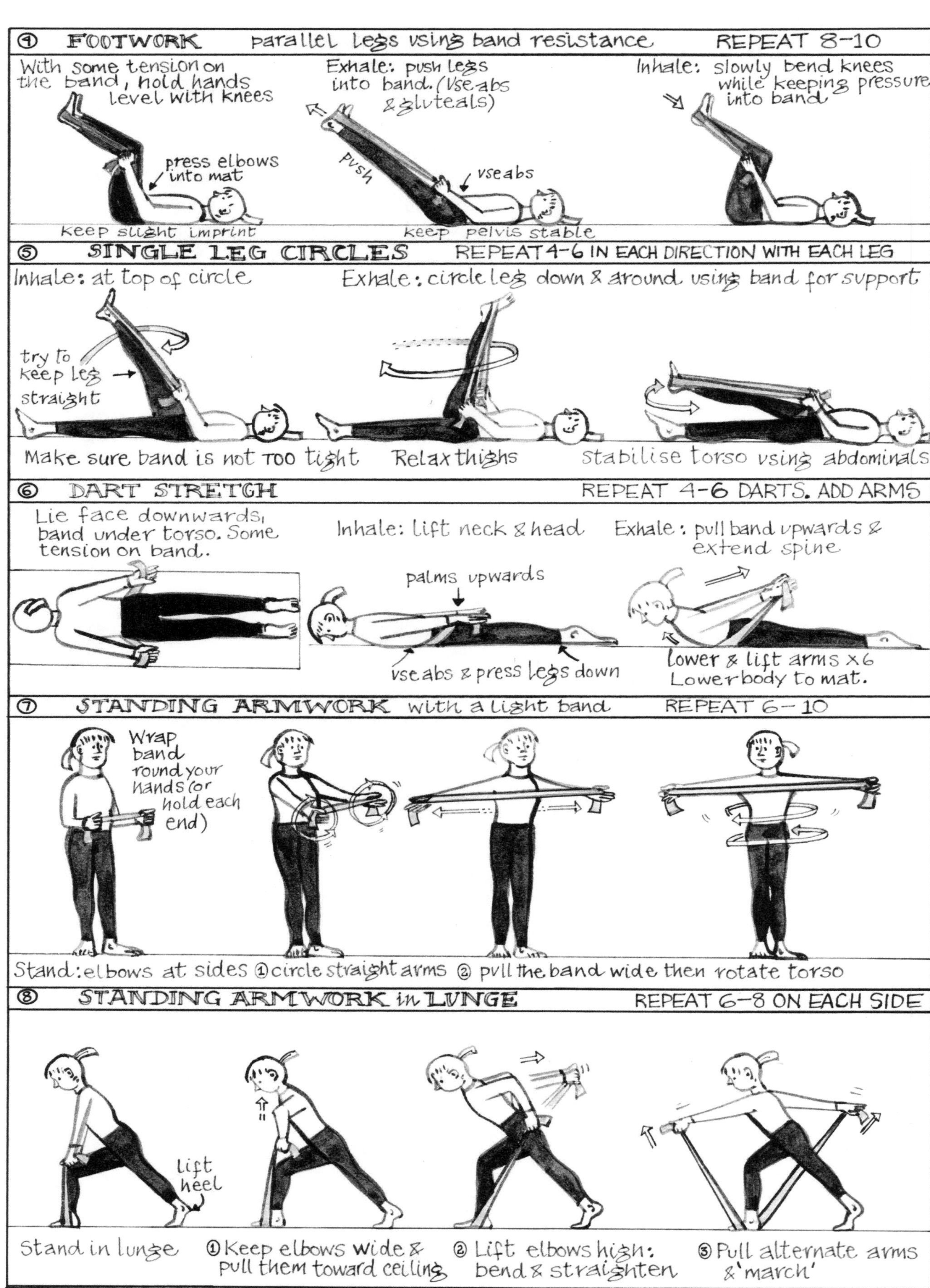
④ FOOTWORK parallel legs using band resistance REPEAT 8-10
With some tension on the band, hold hands level with knees
Exhale: push legs into band. (Use abs & gluteals)
Inhale: slowly bend knees while keeping pressure into band
press elbows into mat
push
use abs
keep slight imprint
keep pelvis stable
⑤ SINGLE LEG CIRCLES REPEAT 4-6 IN EACH DIRECTION WITH EACH LEG
Inhale: at top of circle
Exhale: circle leg down & around using band for support
try to keep leg straight
Make sure band is not too tight
Relax thighs
stabilise torso using abdominals
⑥ DART STRETCH REPEAT 4-6 DARTS. ADD ARMS
Lie face downwards, band under torso. Some tension on band.
Inhale: lift neck & head
Exhale: pull band upwards & extend spine
palms upwards
use abs & press legs down
lower & lift arms x6
Lower body to mat.
⑦ STANDING ARMWORK with a light band REPEAT 6-10
Wrap band round your hands (or hold each end)
Stand: elbows at sides ① circle straight arms ② pull the band wide then rotate torso
⑧ STANDING ARMWORK in LUNGE REPEAT 6-8 ON EACH SIDE
lift heel
Stand in lunge
① Keep elbows wide & pull them toward ceiling
② Lift elbows high: bend & straighten
③ Pull alternate arms & 'march'

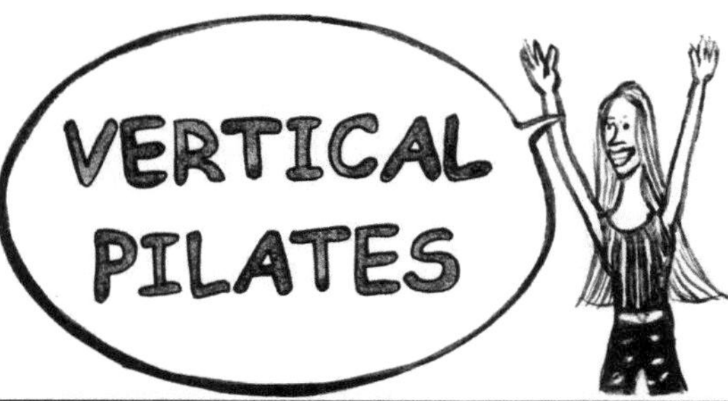

AS A FORMER CONTEMPORARY DANCER LIZ IS PASSIONATE ABOUT TEACHING STANDING PILATES. IN LIFE WE NEED FUNCTIONAL STRENGTH & THREE DIMENSIONAL MOVEMENT THAT CAN ONLY BE ACHIEVED STANDING UPRIGHT. MOST PEOPLE WHO MASTER PILATES HAVE GOOD TRUNK CONTROL BUT FIND STANDING BALANCE CHALLENGING. THIS CLASS IS MODIFIED FROM ONE OF LIZ'S WORKSHOPS.

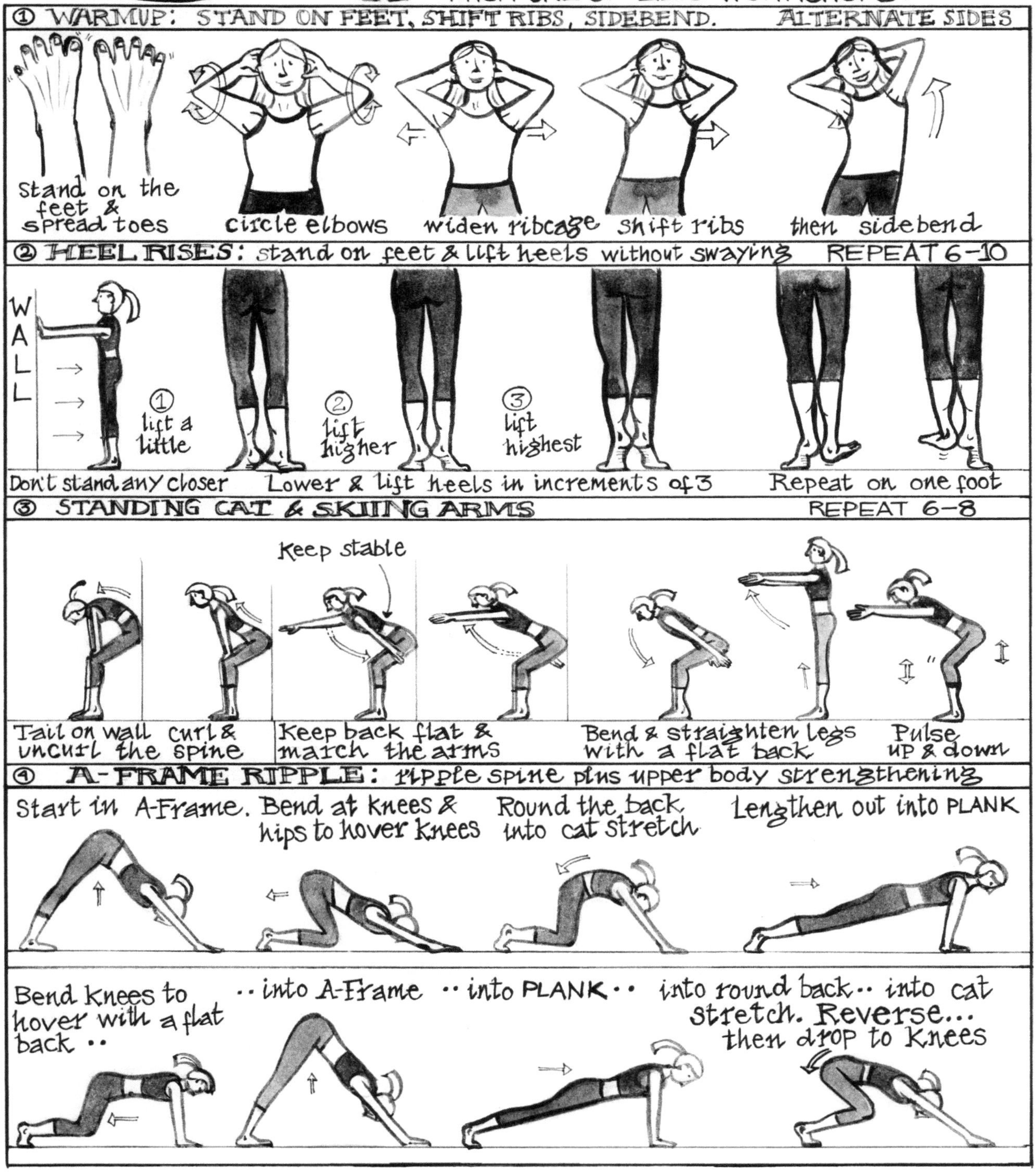

① WARMUP: STAND ON FEET, SHIFT RIBS, SIDEBEND. ALTERNATE SIDES

Stand on the feet & spread toes
circle elbows
widen ribcage
shift ribs
then sidebend

② HEEL RISES: stand on feet & lift heels without swaying REPEAT 6–10

WALL
Don't stand any closer
① lift a little
② lift higher
③ lift highest
Lower & lift heels in increments of 3
Repeat on one foot

③ STANDING CAT & SKIING ARMS REPEAT 6–8

Keep stable
Tail on wall curl & uncurl the spine
Keep back flat & march the arms
Bend & straighten legs with a flat back
Pulse up & down

④ A-FRAME RIPPLE: ripple spine plus upper body strengthening

Start in A-Frame.
Bend at knees & hips to hover knees
Round the back into cat stretch
Lengthen out into PLANK

Bend knees to hover with a flat back ..
.. into A-Frame
.. into PLANK ..
into round back .. into cat stretch. Reverse... then drop to Knees

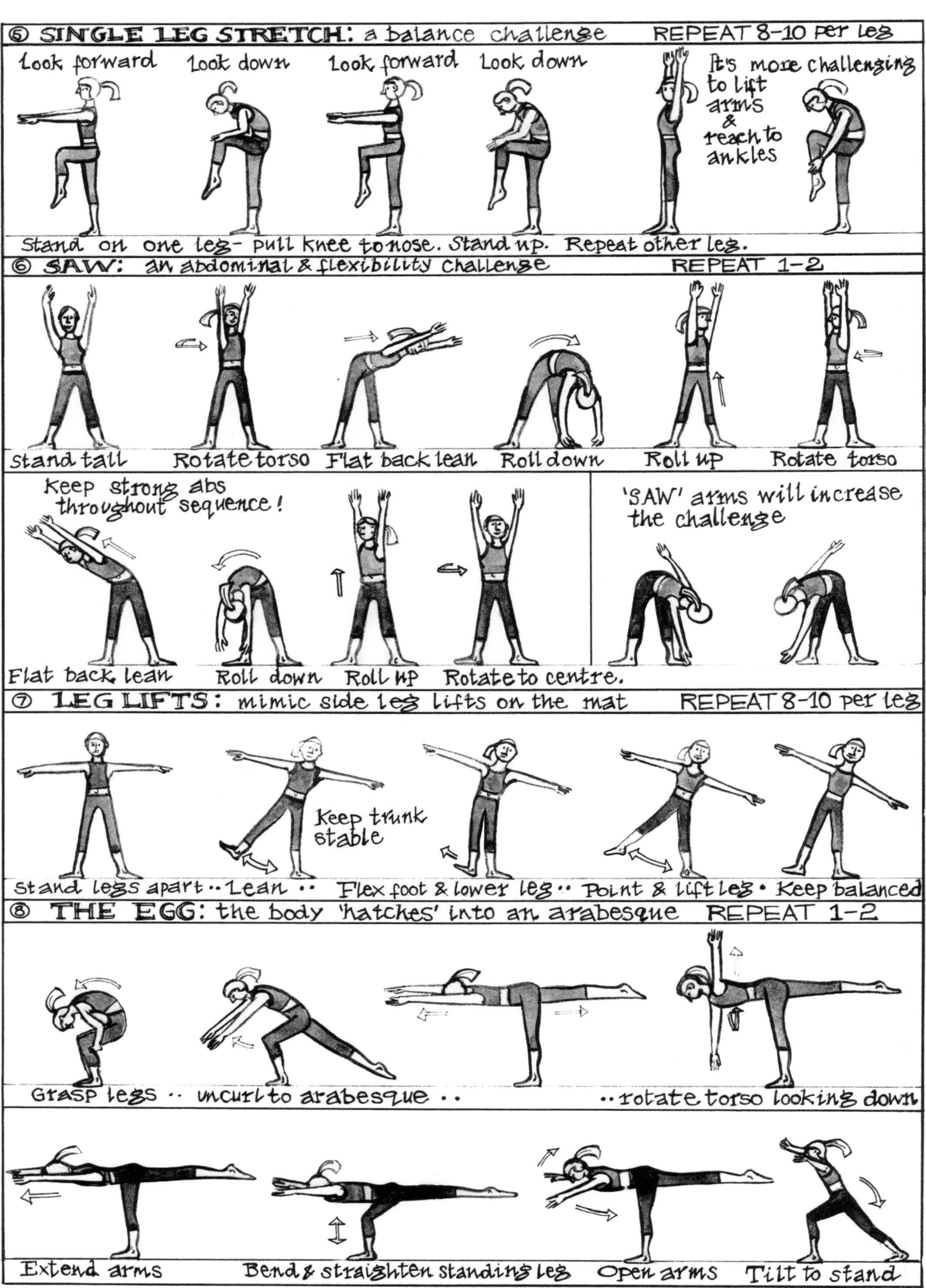
⑤ SINGLE LEG STRETCH: a balance challenge
REPEAT 8-10 per leg
Look forward
Look down
Look forward
Look down
It's more challenging to lift arms & reach to ankles
Stand on one leg- pull knee to nose. Stand up. Repeat other leg.
⑥ SAW: an abdominal & flexibility challenge
REPEAT 1-2
Stand tall
Rotate torso
Flat back lean
Roll down
Roll up
Rotate torso
Keep strong abs throughout sequence!
Flat back lean
Roll down
Roll up
Rotate to centre.
'SAW' arms will increase the challenge
⑦ LEG LIFTS: mimic side leg lifts on the mat
REPEAT 8-10 per leg
Keep trunk stable
Stand legs apart .. Lean .. Flex foot & lower leg .. Point & lift leg • Keep balanced
⑧ THE EGG: the body 'hatches' into an arabesque
REPEAT 1-2
Grasp legs .. uncurl to arabesque ..
.. rotate torso looking down
Extend arms
Bend & straighten standing leg
Open arms
Tilt to stand

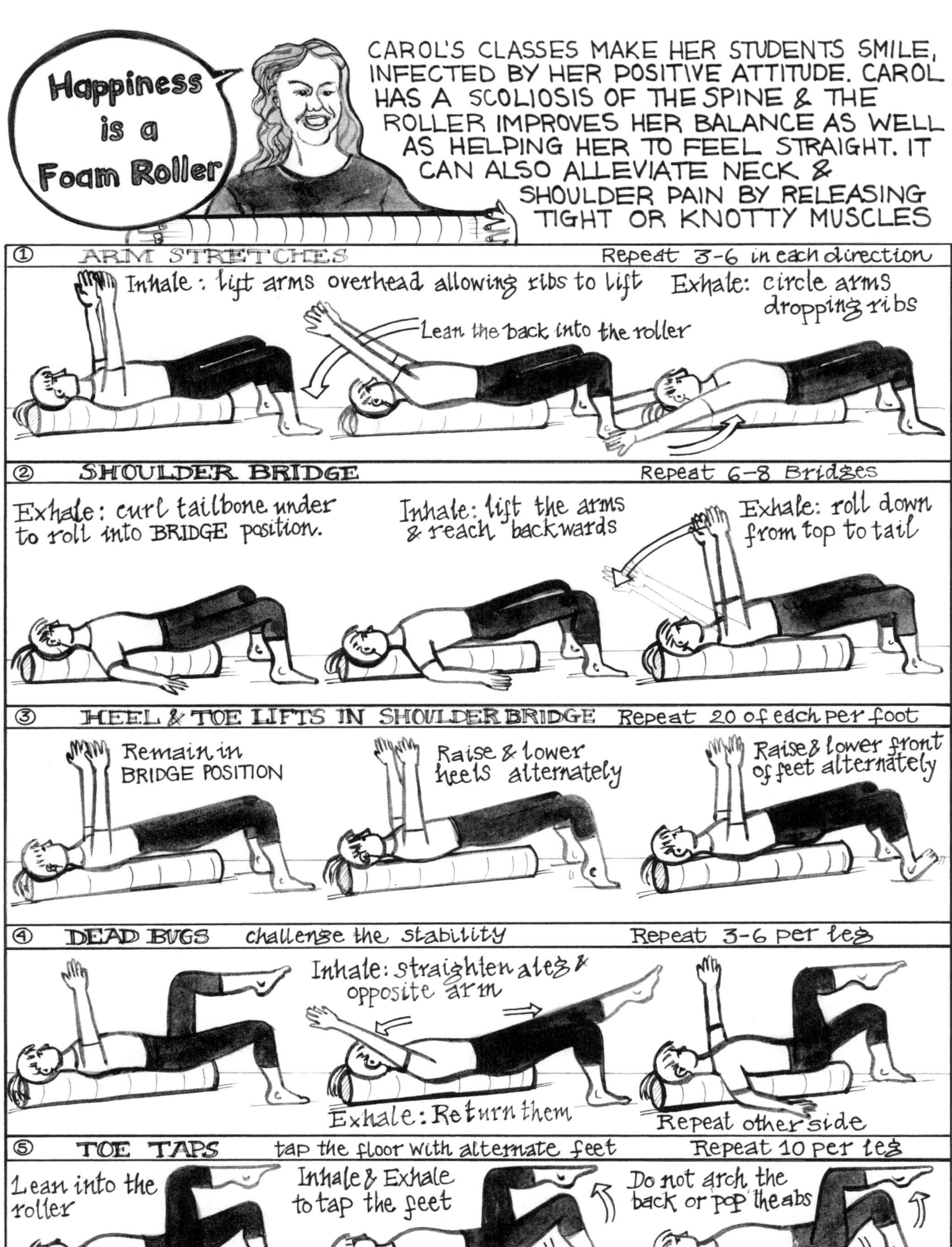
Happiness is a Foam Roller
CAROL'S CLASSES MAKE HER STUDENTS SMILE, INFECTED BY HER POSITIVE ATTITUDE. CAROL HAS A SCOLIOSIS OF THE SPINE & THE ROLLER IMPROVES HER BALANCE AS WELL AS HELPING HER TO FEEL STRAIGHT. IT CAN ALSO ALLEVIATE NECK & SHOULDER PAIN BY RELEASING TIGHT OR KNOTTY MUSCLES
① ARM STRETCHES
Repeat 3-6 in each direction
Inhale: lift arms overhead allowing ribs to lift
Exhale: circle arms dropping ribs
Lean the back into the roller
② SHOULDER BRIDGE
Repeat 6-8 Bridges
Exhale: curl tailbone under to roll into BRIDGE position.
Inhale: lift the arms & reach backwards
Exhale: roll down from top to tail
③ HEEL & TOE LIFTS IN SHOULDER BRIDGE
Repeat 20 of each per foot
Remain in BRIDGE POSITION
Raise & lower heels alternately
Raise & lower front of feet alternately
④ DEAD BUGS
challenge the stability
Repeat 3-6 per leg
Inhale: straighten a leg & opposite arm
Exhale: Return them
Repeat other side
⑤ TOE TAPS
tap the floor with alternate feet
Repeat 10 per leg
Lean into the roller
Inhale & Exhale to tap the feet
Do not arch the back or pop the abs

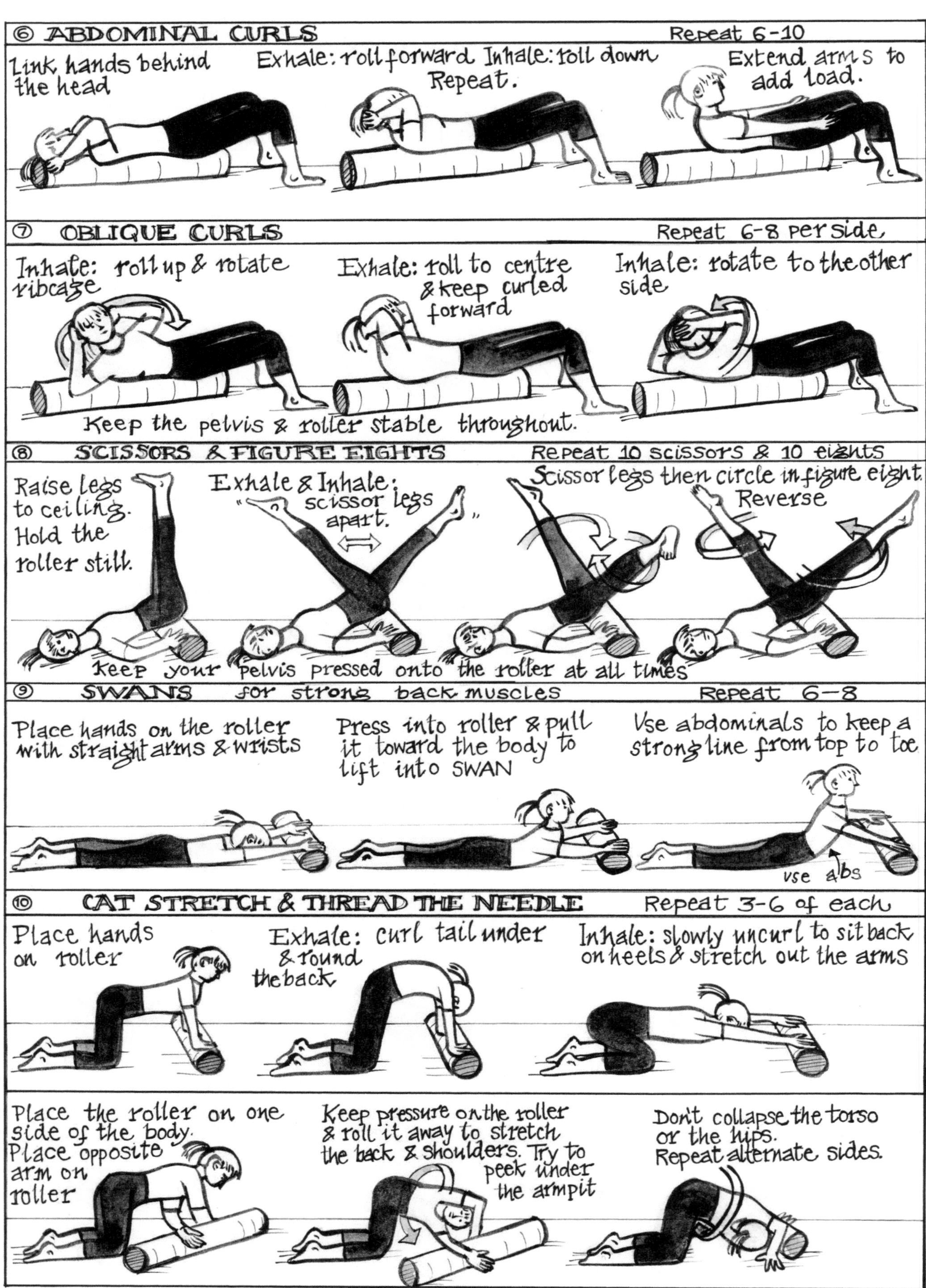

⑥ ABDOMINAL CURLS
Repeat 6-10
Link hands behind the head
Exhale: roll forward Inhale: roll down Repeat.
Extend arms to add load.
⑦ OBLIQUE CURLS
Repeat 6-8 per side
Inhale: roll up & rotate ribcage
Exhale: roll to centre & keep curled forward
Inhale: rotate to the other side
Keep the pelvis & roller stable throughout.
⑧ SCISSORS & FIGURE EIGHTS
Repeat 10 scissors & 10 eights
Raise legs to ceiling. Hold the roller still.
Exhale & Inhale: "scissor legs apart."
Scissor legs then circle in figure eight.
Reverse
Keep your pelvis pressed onto the roller at all times
⑨ SWANS for strong back muscles
Repeat 6-8
Place hands on the roller with straight arms & wrists
Press into roller & pull it toward the body to lift into SWAN
Use abdominals to keep a strong line from top to toe
use abs
⑩ CAT STRETCH & THREAD THE NEEDLE
Repeat 3-6 of each
Place hands on roller
Exhale: curl tail under & round the back
Inhale: slowly uncurl to sit back on heels & stretch out the arms
Place the roller on one side of the body. Place opposite arm on roller
Keep pressure on the roller & roll it away to stretch the back & shoulders. Try to peek under the armpit
Don't collapse the torso or the hips. Repeat alternate sides.

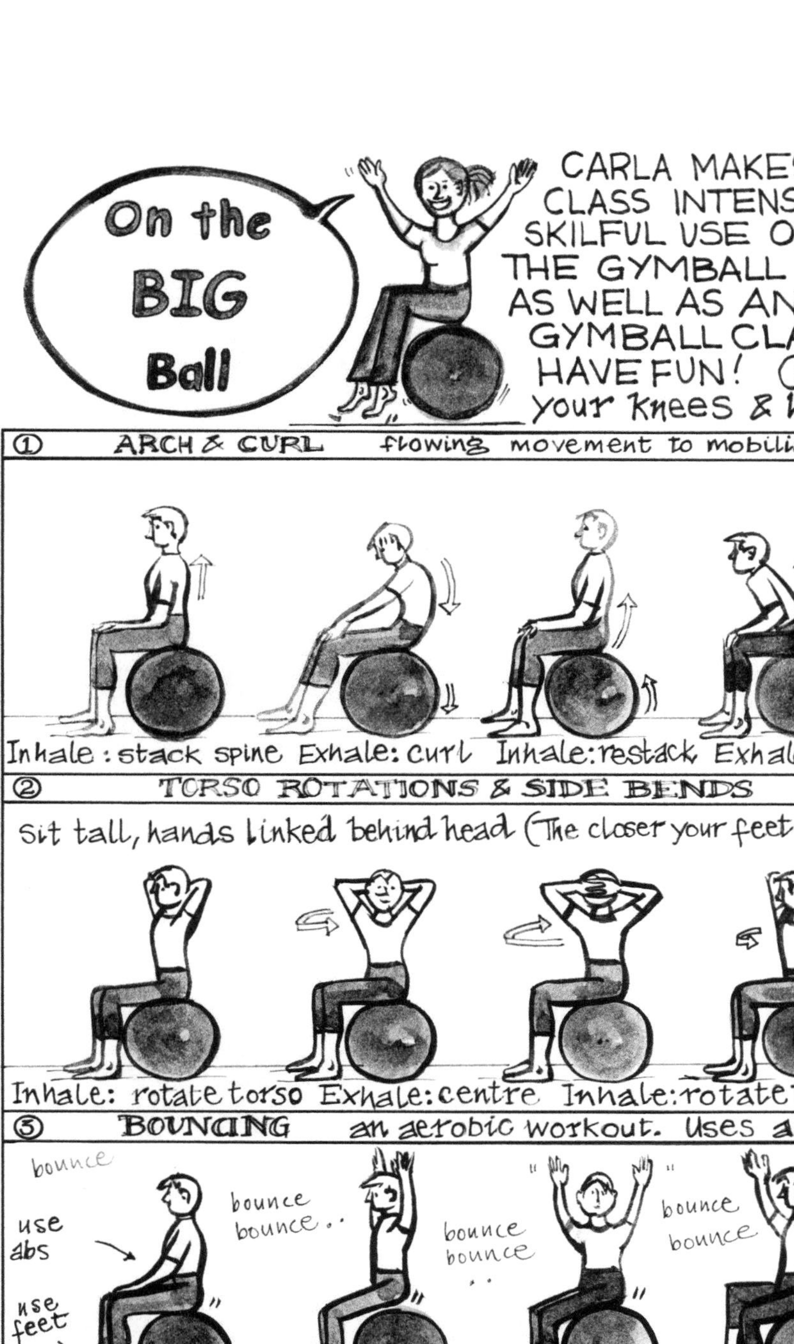

On the BIG Ball

CARLA MAKES THE SIMPLEST PILATES CLASS INTENSE & STIMULATING WITH HER SKILFUL USE OF RICH & VARIED CUEING. THE GYMBALL ADDS A BALANCE CHALLENGE AS WELL AS AN AEROBIC WORKOUT. CARLA'S GYMBALL CLASS IS STRONG & ENERGETIC HAVE FUN! (Seated on the correct sized ball your knees & hips will be at 90 degrees)

① ARCH & CURL

flowing movement to mobilise the spine — REPEAT 6-10

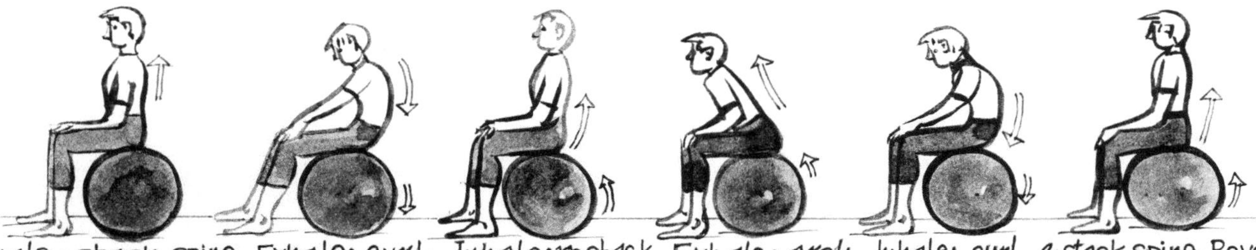

Inhale: stack spine Exhale: curl Inhale: restack Exhale: arch Inhale: curl & stack spine. Reverse

② TORSO ROTATIONS & SIDE BENDS

REPEAT 3-6

Sit tall, hands linked behind head (The closer your feet are together, the more difficult this is)

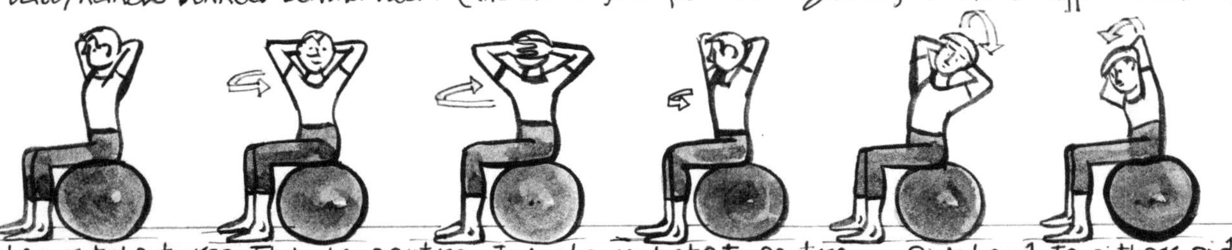

Inhale: rotate torso Exhale: centre Inhale: rotate to centre. Sidebend to either side

③ BOUNCING

an aerobic workout. Uses abs & legs — Bounce till you tire!

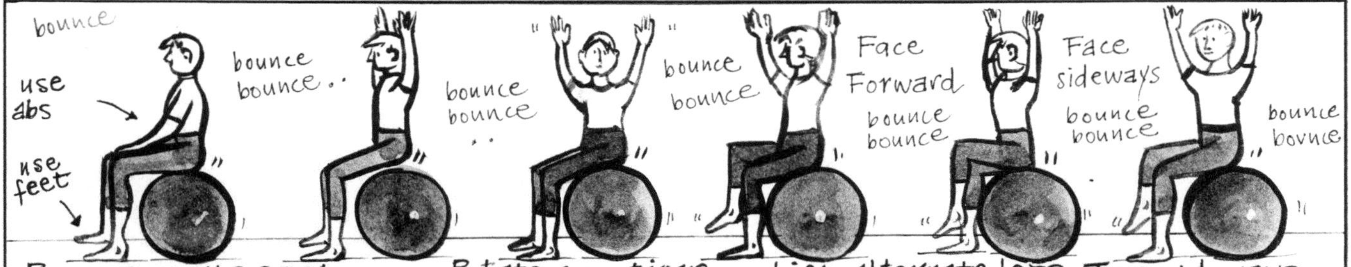

bounce
use abs
use feet
bounce bounce..
bounce bounce
bounce bounce
Face Forward
bounce bounce
Face sideways
bounce bounce
bounce bounce

Bounce on the spot. Rotate & continue. Lift alternate legs. Face sideways

④ BRIDGE ON THE BALL

REPEAT 6-8

Lie with knees bent over the ball

Exhale: straighten legs & role hips up into the BRIDGE
Inhale: lift arms

Exhale: roll spine onto mat
Inhale: lower arms

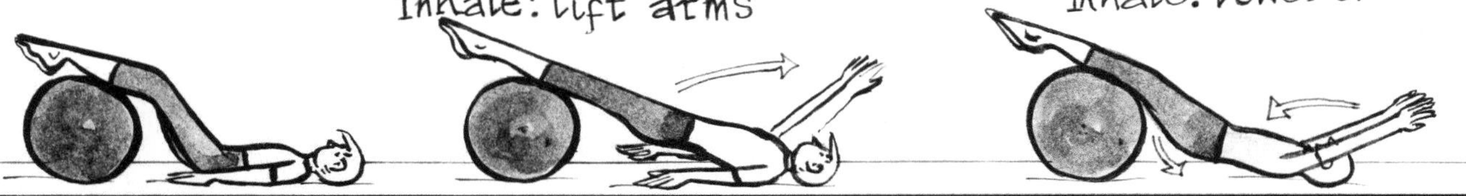

⑤ SEMICIRCLE

works hamstrings — REPEAT 3-4 in each direction

Bend knees. Place soles of feet on top of ball

Exhale: press into ball & lift hips

Inhale: hold position
Exhale: roll ball so legs straighten then roll down
Reverse

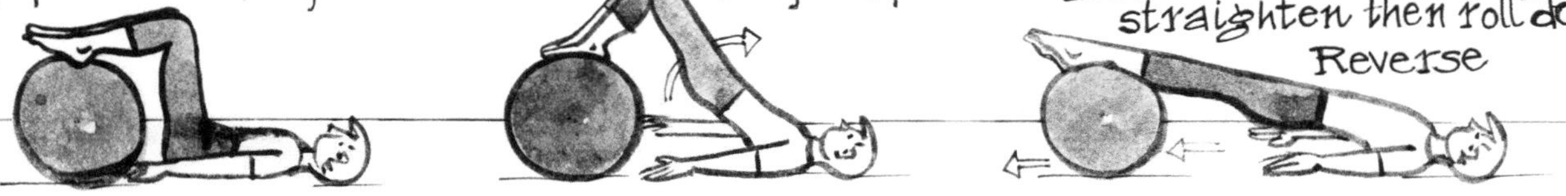

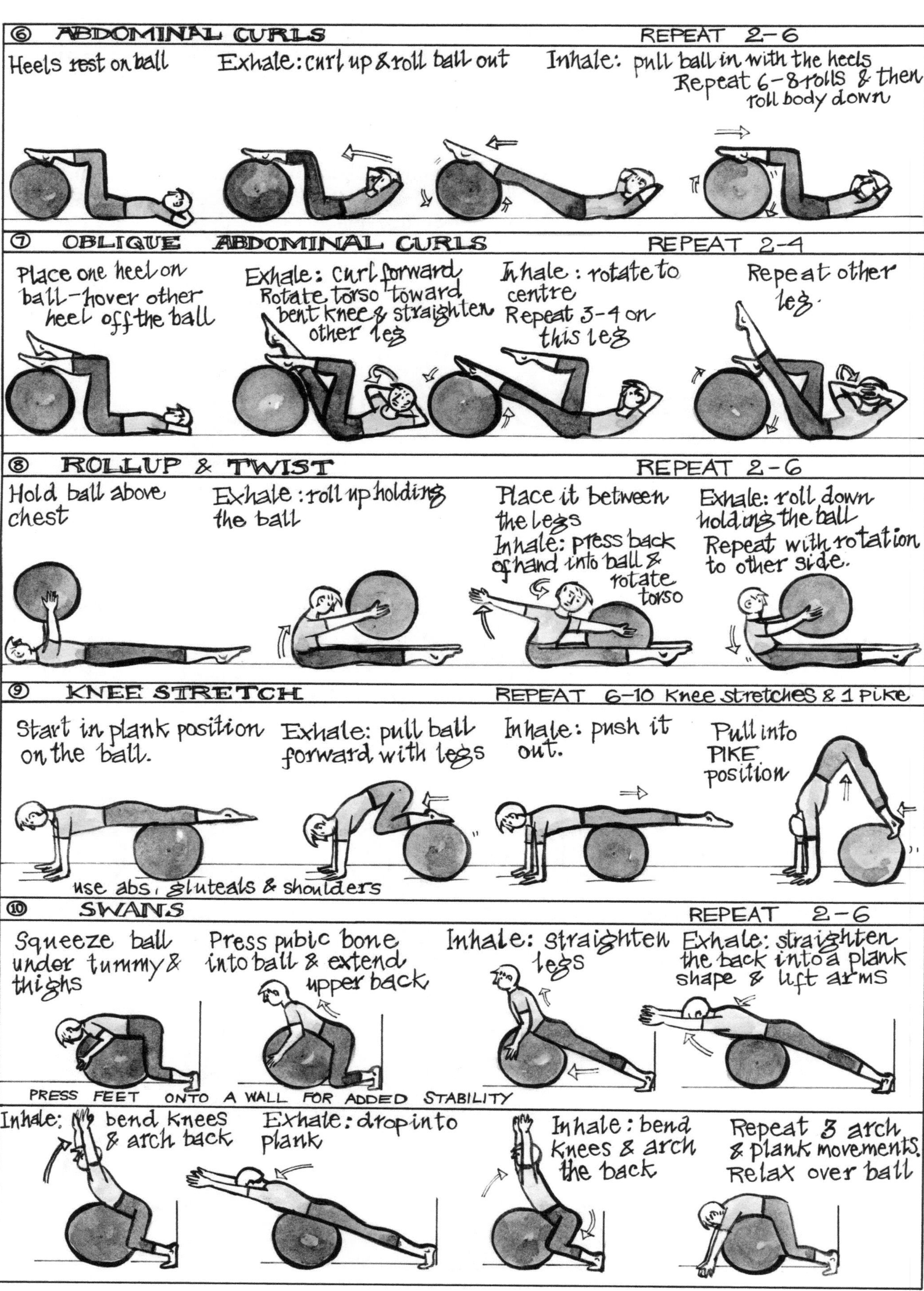
⑥ ABDOMINAL CURLS
REPEAT 2–6
Heels rest on ball
Exhale: curl up & roll ball out
Inhale: pull ball in with the heels
Repeat 6–8 rolls & then roll body down
⑦ OBLIQUE ABDOMINAL CURLS
REPEAT 2-4
Place one heel on ball – hover other heel off the ball
Exhale: curl forward Rotate torso toward bent knee & straighten other leg
Inhale: rotate to centre Repeat 3–4 on this leg
Repeat other leg.
⑧ ROLLUP & TWIST
REPEAT 2–6
Hold ball above chest
Exhale: roll up holding the ball
Place it between the legs Inhale: press back of hand into ball & rotate torso
Exhale: roll down holding the ball Repeat with rotation to other side.
⑨ KNEE STRETCH
REPEAT 6–10 knee stretches & 1 pike
Start in plank position on the ball.
Exhale: pull ball forward with legs
Inhale: push it out.
Pull into PIKE position
use abs, gluteals & shoulders
⑩ SWANS
REPEAT 2–6
Squeeze ball under tummy & thighs
Press pubic bone into ball & extend upper back
Inhale: straighten legs
Exhale: straighten the back into a plank shape & lift arms
PRESS FEET ONTO A WALL FOR ADDED STABILITY
Inhale: bend knees & arch back
Exhale: drop into plank
Inhale: bend knees & arch the back
Repeat 3 arch & plank movements. Relax over ball

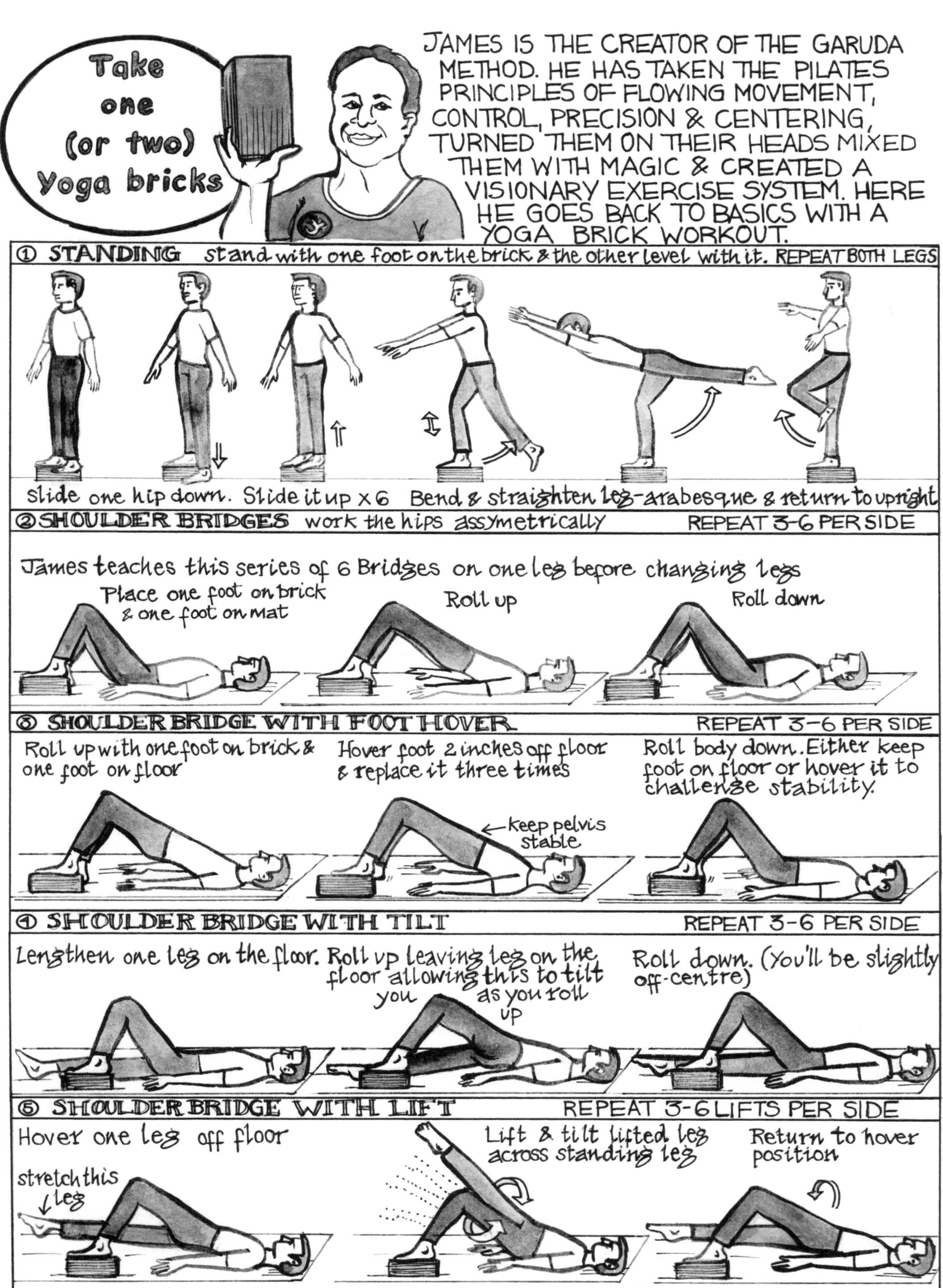

Take one (or two) yoga bricks
JAMES IS THE CREATOR OF THE GARUDA METHOD. HE HAS TAKEN THE PILATES PRINCIPLES OF FLOWING MOVEMENT, CONTROL, PRECISION & CENTERING, TURNED THEM ON THEIR HEADS MIXED THEM WITH MAGIC & CREATED A VISIONARY EXERCISE SYSTEM. HERE HE GOES BACK TO BASICS WITH A YOGA BRICK WORKOUT.
① STANDING stand with one foot on the brick & the other level with it. REPEAT BOTH LEGS
slide one hip down. Slide it up x 6 Bend & straighten leg - arabesque & return to upright
② SHOULDER BRIDGES work the hips assymetrically REPEAT 3-6 PER SIDE
James teaches this series of 6 Bridges on one leg before changing legs
Place one foot on brick & one foot on mat
Roll up
Roll down
③ SHOULDER BRIDGE WITH FOOT HOVER REPEAT 3-6 PER SIDE
Roll up with one foot on brick & one foot on floor
Hover foot 2 inches off floor & replace it three times
Roll body down. Either keep foot on floor or hover it to challenge stability.
keep pelvis stable
④ SHOULDER BRIDGE WITH TILT REPEAT 3-6 PER SIDE
Lengthen one leg on the floor.
Roll up leaving leg on the floor allowing this to tilt you as you roll up
Roll down. (You'll be slightly off-centre)
⑤ SHOULDER BRIDGE WITH LIFT REPEAT 3-6 LIFTS PER SIDE
Hover one leg off floor
stretch this leg
Lift & tilt lifted leg across standing leg
Return to hover position

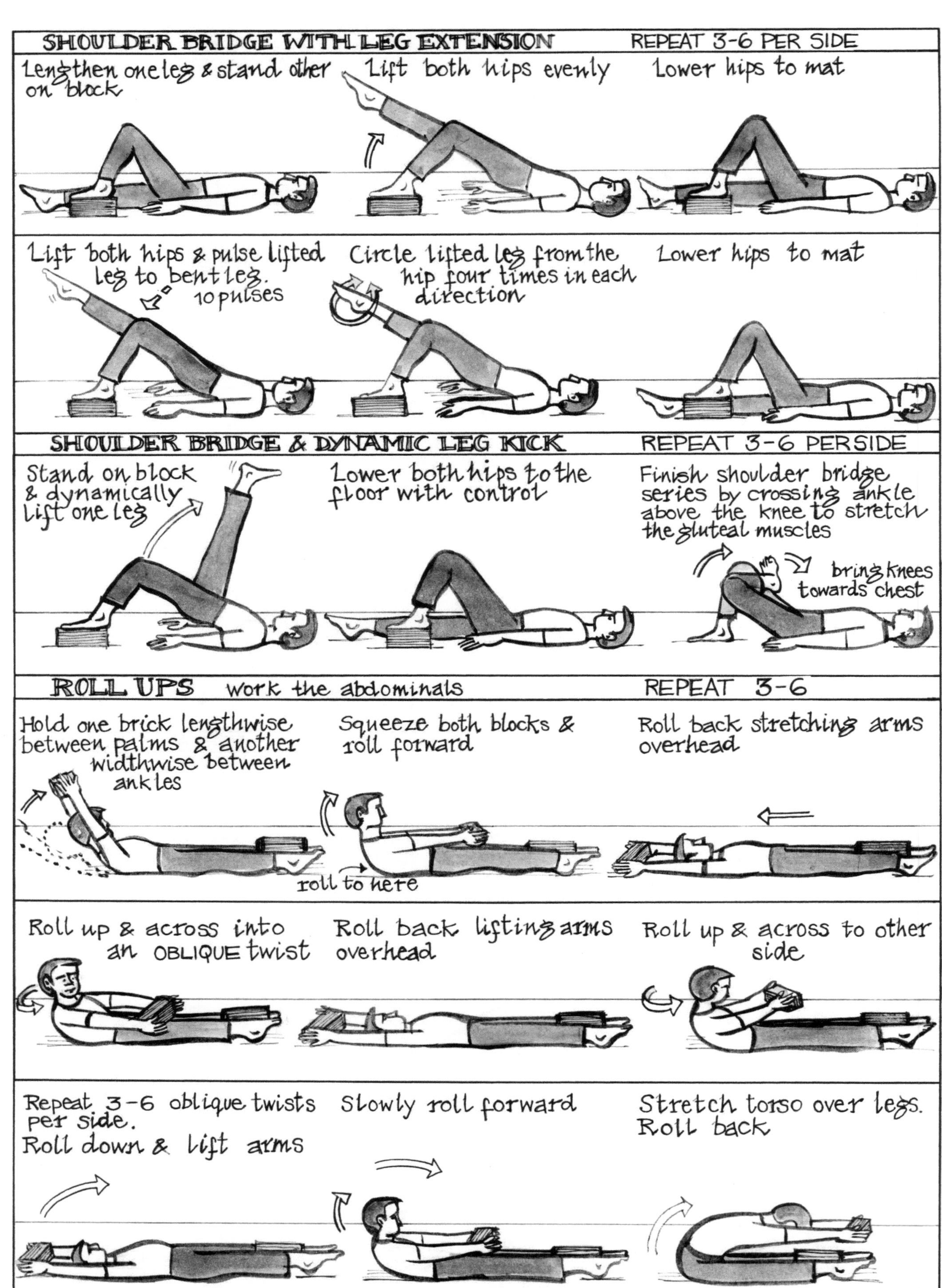
SHOULDER BRIDGE WITH LEG EXTENSION
REPEAT 3-6 PER SIDE
Lengthen one leg & stand other on block
Lift both hips evenly
Lower hips to mat
Lift both hips & pulse lifted leg to bent leg.
10 pulses
Circle lifted leg from the hip four times in each direction
Lower hips to mat
SHOULDER BRIDGE & DYNAMIC LEG KICK
REPEAT 3-6 PERSIDE
Stand on block & dynamically lift one leg
Lower both hips to the floor with control
Finish shoulder bridge series by crossing ankle above the knee to stretch the gluteal muscles
bring knees towards chest
ROLL UPS
work the abdominals
REPEAT 3-6
Hold one brick lengthwise between palms & another widthwise between ankles
Squeeze both blocks & roll forward
Roll back stretching arms overhead
roll to here
Roll up & across into an OBLIQUE twist
Roll back lifting arms overhead
Roll up & across to other side
Repeat 3-6 oblique twists per side.
Roll down & lift arms
Slowly roll forward
Stretch torso over legs.
Roll back

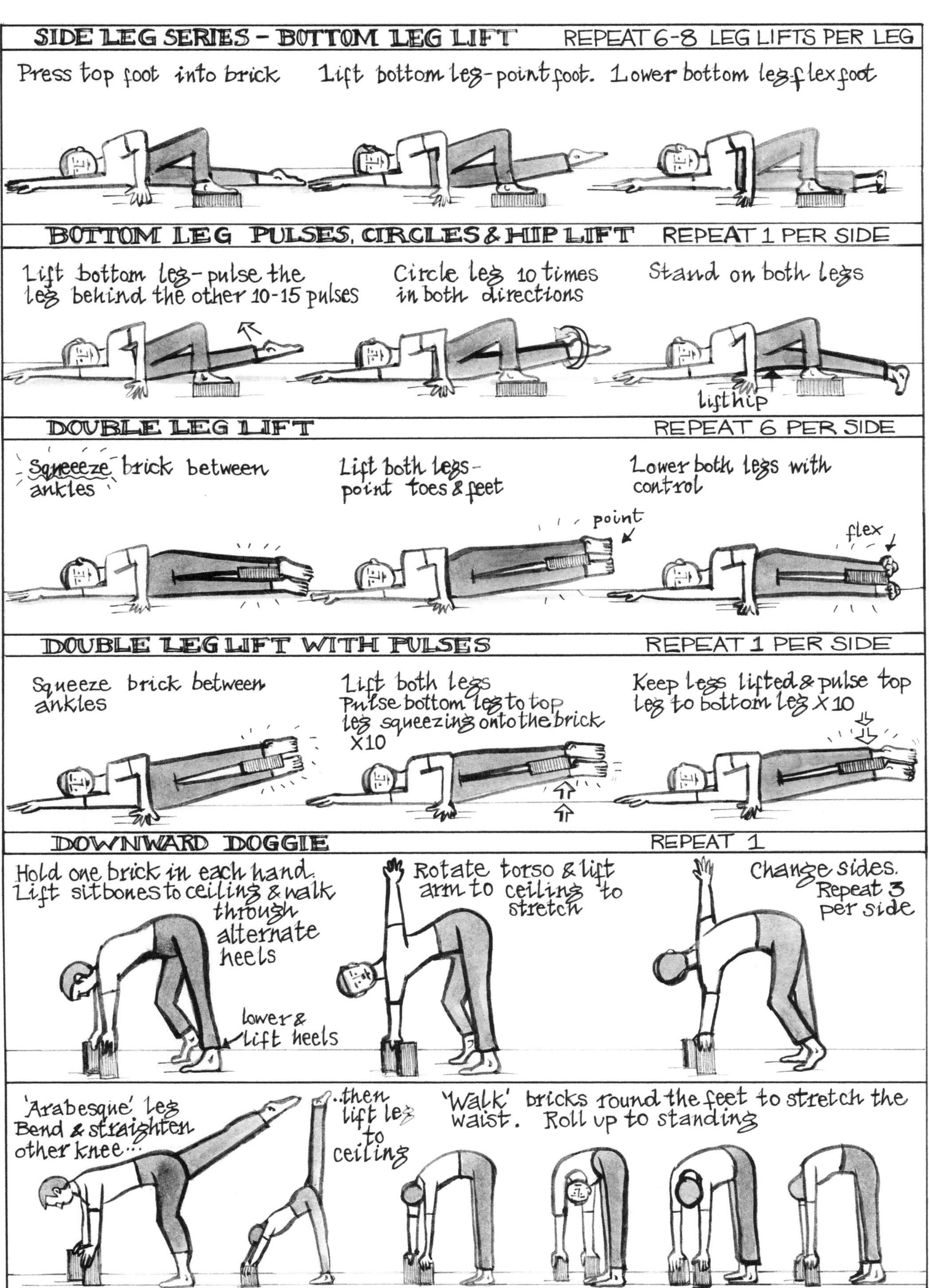
SIDE LEG SERIES – BOTTOM LEG LIFT
REPEAT 6-8 LEG LIFTS PER LEG
Press top foot into brick
Lift bottom leg-point foot.
Lower bottom leg-flex foot
BOTTOM LEG PULSES, CIRCLES & HIP LIFT
REPEAT 1 PER SIDE
Lift bottom leg-pulse the leg behind the other 10-15 pulses
Circle leg 10 times in both directions
Stand on both legs
lift hip
DOUBLE LEG LIFT
REPEAT 6 PER SIDE
Squeeze brick between ankles
Lift both legs-point toes & feet
Lower both legs with control
point
flex
DOUBLE LEG LIFT WITH PULSES
REPEAT 1 PER SIDE
Squeeze brick between ankles
Lift both legs Pulse bottom leg to top leg squeezing onto the brick x10
Keep legs lifted & pulse top leg to bottom leg x 10
DOWNWARD DOGGIE
REPEAT 1
Hold one brick in each hand. Lift sitbones to ceiling & walk through alternate heels
lower & lift heels
Rotate torso & lift arm to ceiling to stretch
Change sides. Repeat 3 per side
'Arabesque' leg Bend & straighten other knee...
..then lift leg to ceiling
'Walk' bricks round the feet to stretch the waist. Roll up to standing

High Performance Hips

SUZANNE IS A MASTER MOVEMENT TRAINER & ANATOMIST WHOSE REPUTATION TRAVELS BEFORE HER. MUCH OF HER TIME IS SPENT RESOLVING MOVEMENT PROBLEMS OF PREMIER LEAGUE FOOTBALL PLAYERS WHOSE HIPS COME UNDER GREAT STRAIN. THESE SEEMINGLY SIMPLE EXERCISES ARE TRIED & TESTED TO ACHIEVE HIP STRENGTH & MOBILITY.

THE OYSTER SERIES

REPEAT EACH 6–10 PER SIDE

DIALLING THROUGH THE HIPS

increases range of movement in the hip

Press top heel on the mat behind bottom heel

Rotate leg from heel to top of thigh

Rotate downwards & upwards pressing heel firmly, aiming to increase movement upwards

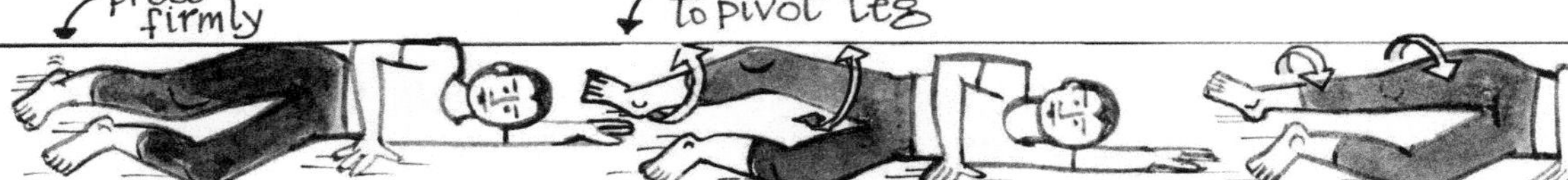

DIAL BOTTOM LEG

Keep top leg still & lift bottom leg

Roll hips back slightly so no longer stacked. Lift top knee & hold position

Rotate bottom leg to top leg & squeeze legs together

Rotate bottom leg to mat.

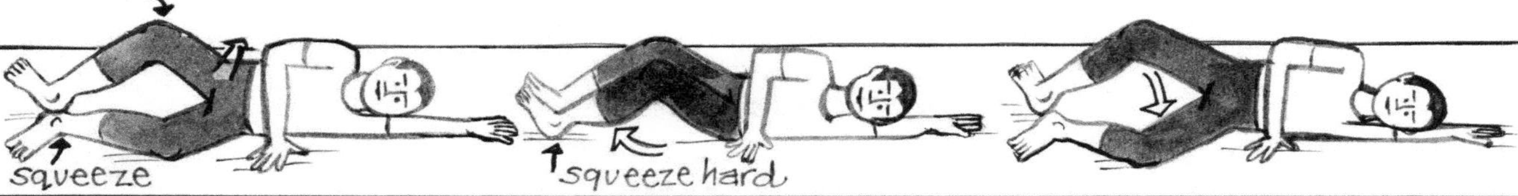

DIAL BOTH LEGS FROM FLOOR

Keep hips rolled back. Create a sensation of bottom leg resisting & top leg pressing

Press heels together & rotate BOTH knees to ceiling

Keep heels squeezed & rotate legs to the mat

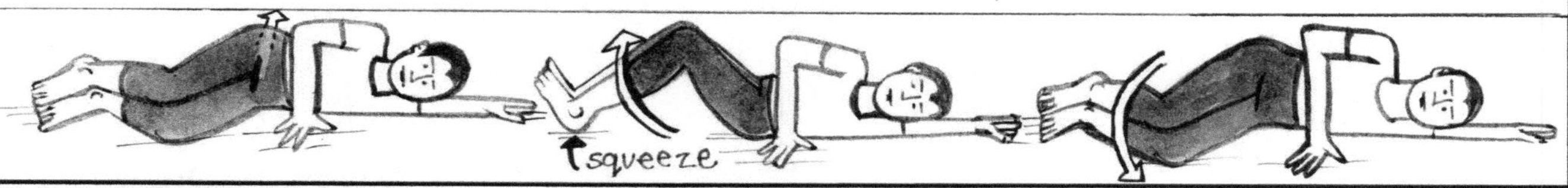

HOVER THE HIPS & ROTATE BOTH LEGS

Press into hand & elbow to hover knees & hips

Press legs together & pivot knees to ceiling

Pivot knees to return. Do not collapse torso.

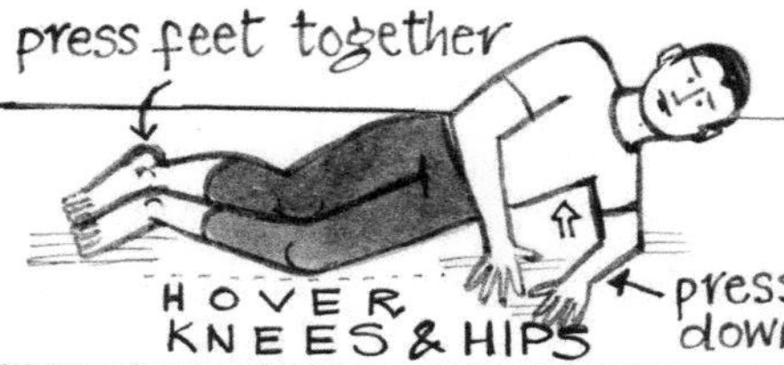

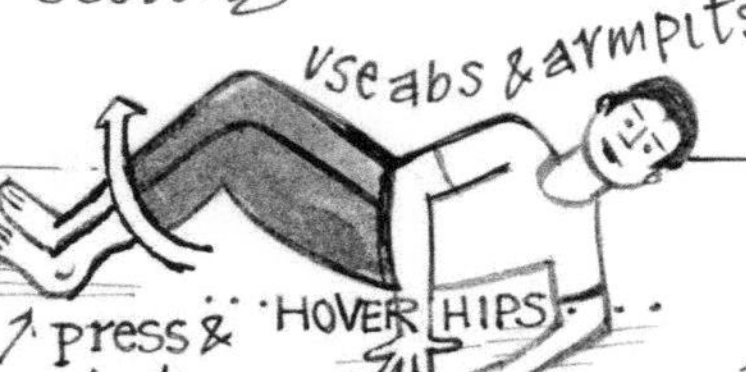

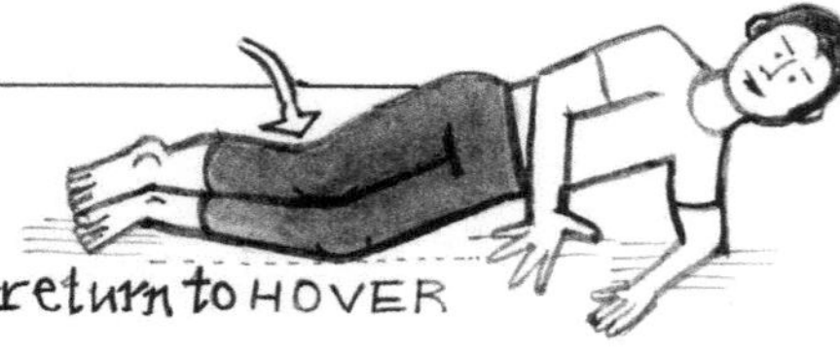

CENTERING THE HIPS — Gently re-educate the deep hip muscles

Place ankle on ball. Press into ball & roll it away until the hip slides down

'Suck' leg into hip socket to draw hip back using deep abdominals.

Draw hip up a little further before slowly releasing tension

Overworking hip, back & thigh muscles can cause hip pain. This aims to calm them.

SINGLE LEG ROTATION IN EXTENSION — REPEAT 6-8 PER LEG

Bend leg at the knee flex the foot, stabilise torso

Lift knee Rotate thigh towards opposite leg

Rotate it to centre

Keep stable

keep stable

ELBOW PLANK GLIDE — connects hips & torso — REPEAT 4-6

Engage abs & shoulders Press from palm to elbow into mat. (Connect arms & shoulders to torso.)

Press & lift body dynamically Use shoulders, abs & gluteals to support plank.

Glide body forward & back 3-4 times Lower body to mat

toes tucked

use shoulders-abs-gluteals

PLANK

WALKING BRIDGE — increases posterior hip efficiency — REPEAT 8-12 PER SIDE

Stand in single leg BRIDGE position with hips level

Glide hips to side of lifted leg & correct balance by standing onto this leg

Lift other leg & repeat this side

Aim to keep hips level & not collapse either side as you sway & use standing heel & foot.

DIPPING BRIDGE — increases hip strength — REPEAT 8-12 PER SIDE

Stand in single leg BRIDGE position with hips level

Drop SUPPORT side of bridge to lose tension

Push support foot into floor to lift hips & level them. (Maintain tone in abs)

use heel

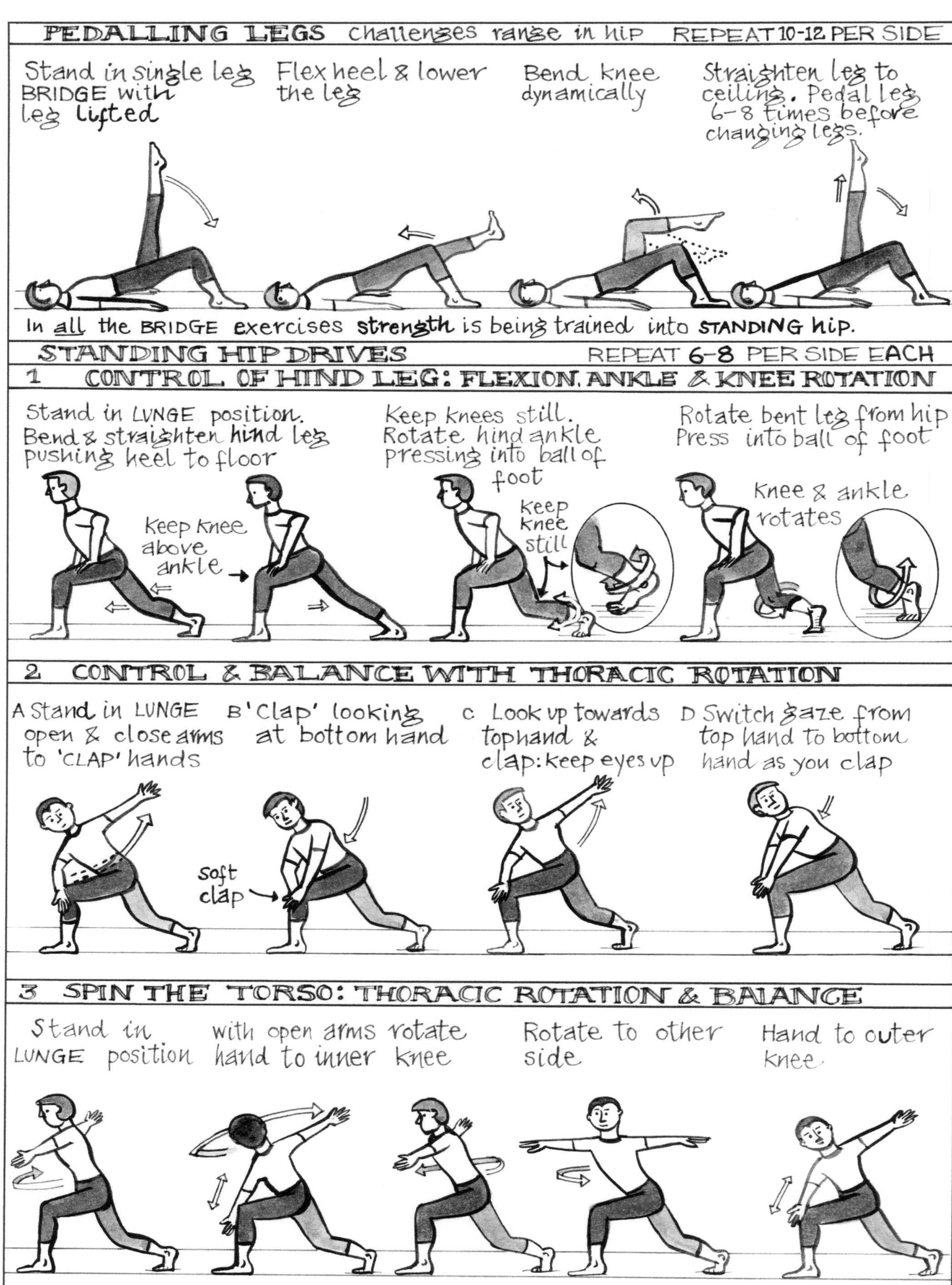
PEDALLING LEGS challenges range in hip REPEAT 10-12 PER SIDE
Stand in single leg BRIDGE with leg lifted
Flex heel & lower the leg
Bend knee dynamically
Straighten leg to ceiling. Pedal leg 6-8 times before changing legs.
In all the BRIDGE exercises strength is being trained into STANDING hip.
STANDING HIP DRIVES REPEAT 6-8 PER SIDE EACH
1 CONTROL OF HIND LEG: FLEXION, ANKLE & KNEE ROTATION
Stand in LUNGE position. Bend & straighten hind leg pushing heel to floor
Keep knee above ankle
Keep knees still. Rotate hind ankle pressing into ball of foot
Keep knee still
Rotate bent leg from hip Press into ball of foot
Knee & ankle rotates
2 CONTROL & BALANCE WITH THORACIC ROTATION
A Stand in LUNGE open & close arms to 'CLAP' hands
B 'Clap' looking at bottom hand
soft clap
C Look up towards top hand & clap: keep eyes up
D Switch gaze from top hand to bottom hand as you clap
3 SPIN THE TORSO: THORACIC ROTATION & BALANCE
Stand in LUNGE position
with open arms rotate hand to inner knee
Rotate to other side
Hand to outer knee

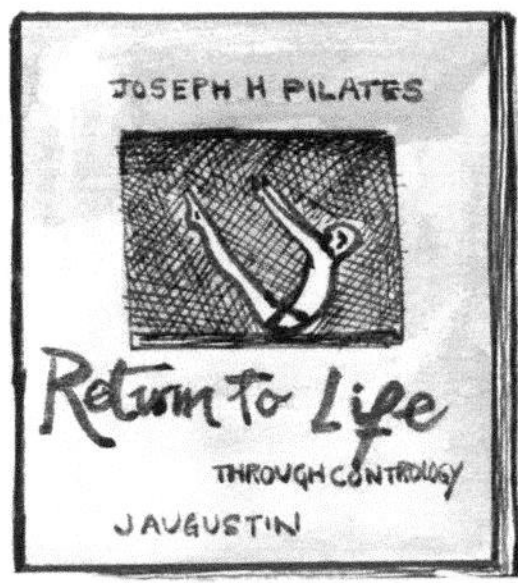

Joseph's Original Sequence

JH Pilates book RETURN TO LIFE THROUGH CONTROLOGY was published in 1945 & contains his 34 original mat exercises & the sequence in which they were taught. Each of these exercises, as well as many modifications is covered in the previous pages.

Exercise				
1 THE HUNDRED				
2 THE ROLL-UP				
3 THE ROLL-OVER				
4 THE SINGLE LEG CIRCLE				
5 ROLLING LIKE A BALL				
6 THE SINGLE LEG STRETCH				
7 THE DOUBLE LEG STRETCH				
8 THE SPINE STRETCH				
9 THE OPEN LEG ROCKER				
10 THE CORKSCREW				
11 THE SAW				
12 THE SWAN DIVE				
13 THE SINGLE LEG KICK				
14 THE DOUBLE LEG KICK				
15 THE NECK PULL				
16 THE SCISSORS				

17 THE BICYCLE	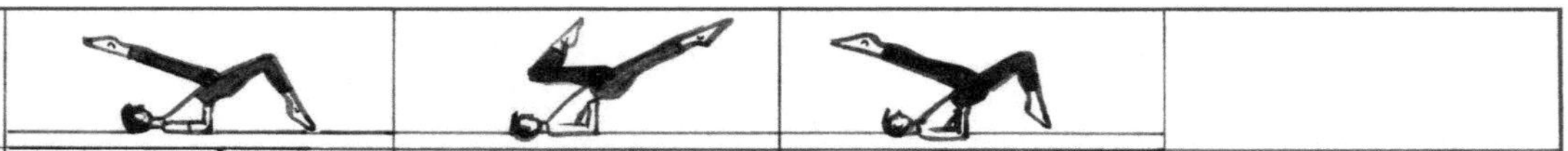
18 THE SHOULDER BRIDGE	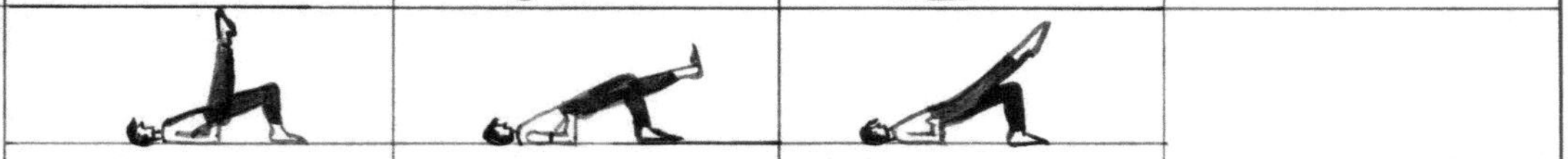
19 THE SPINE TWIST	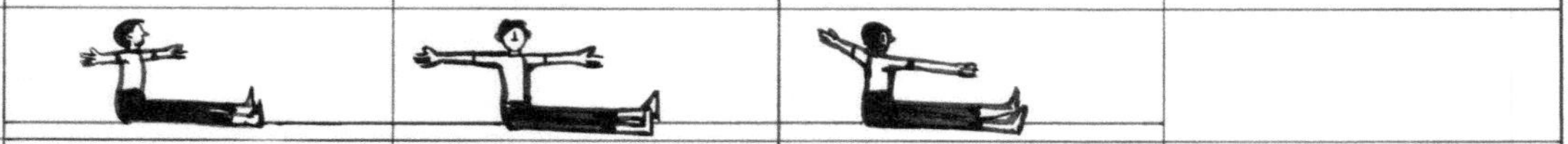
20 THE JACK KNIFE	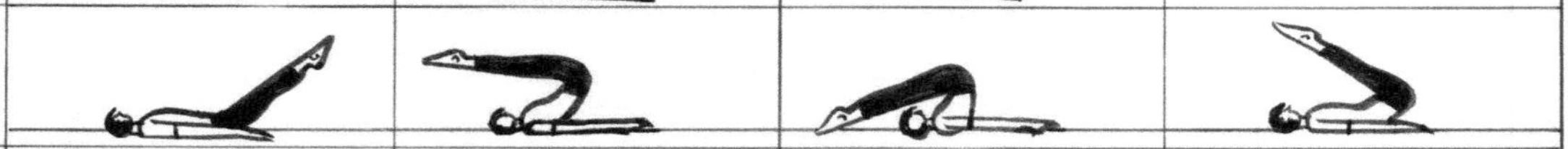
21 THE SIDE KICK	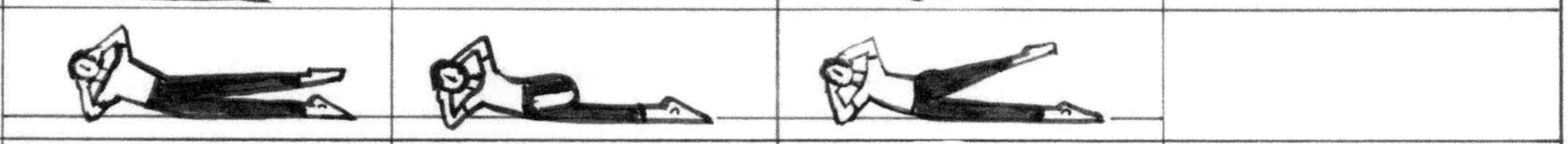
22 THE TEASER	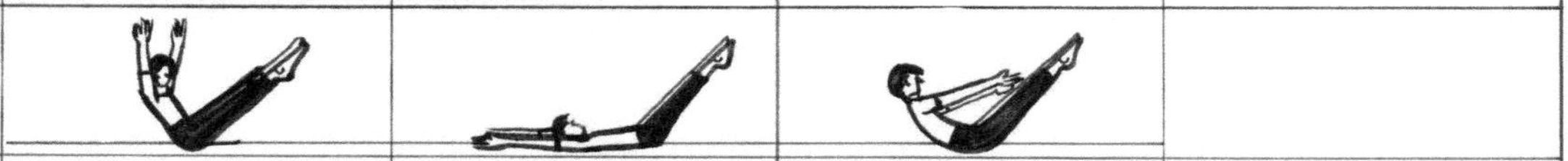
23 THE HIP TWIST	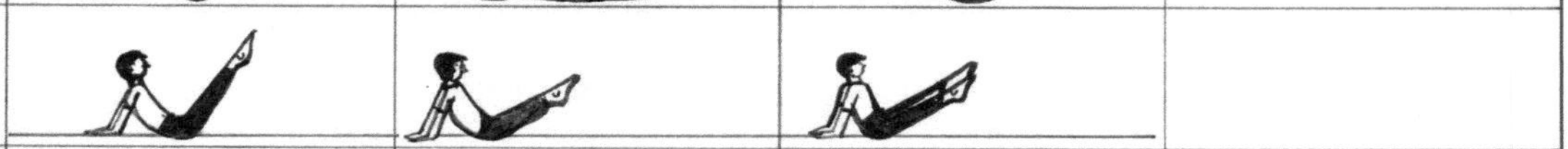
24 SWIMMING	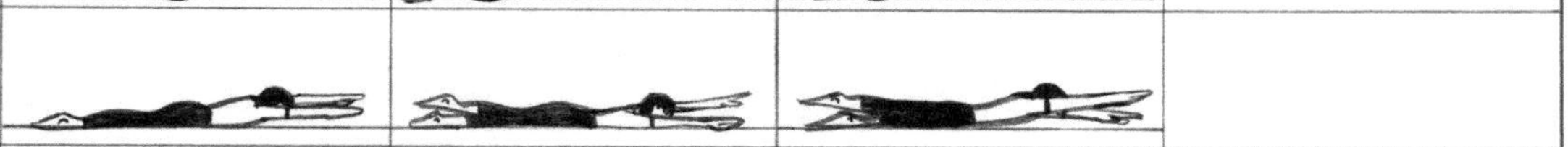
25 THE LEG-PULL FRONT	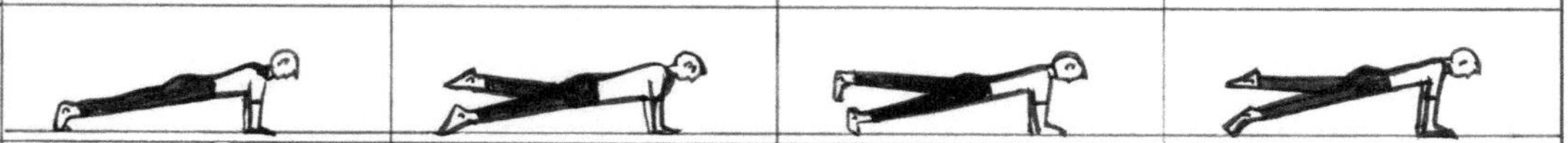
26 THE LEG-PULL	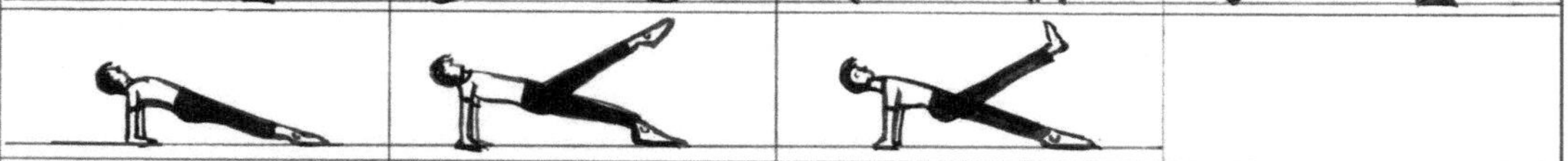
27 THE SIDE-KICK KNEELING	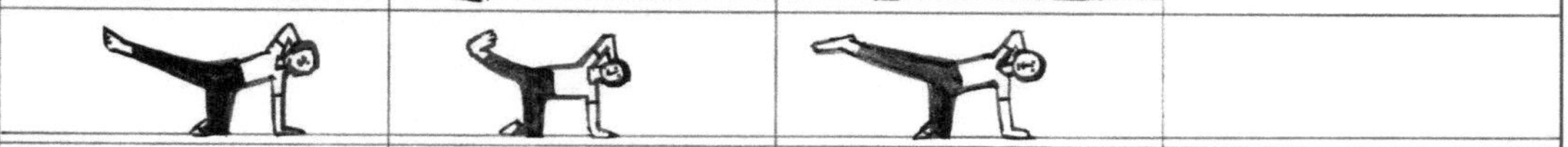
28 THE SIDE BEND	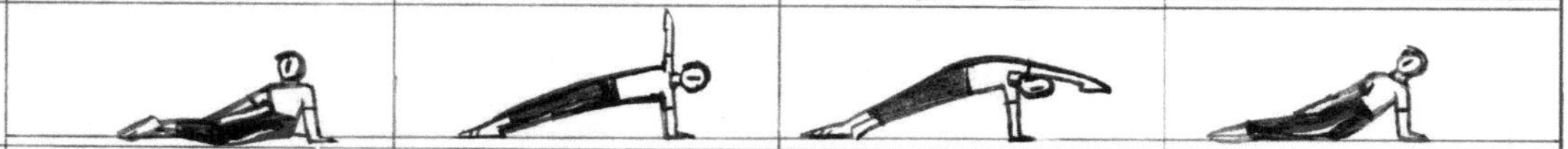
29 THE BOOMERANG	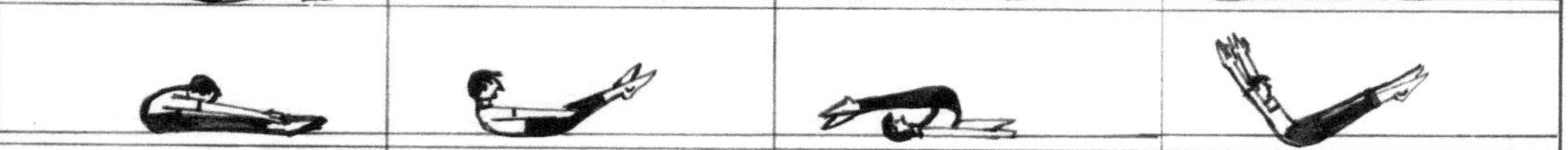
30 THE SEAL	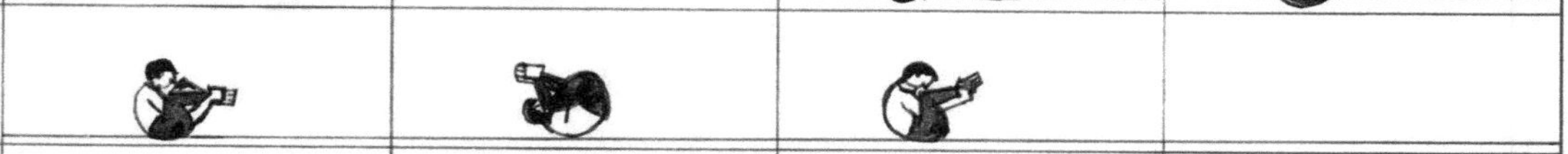
31 THE CRAB	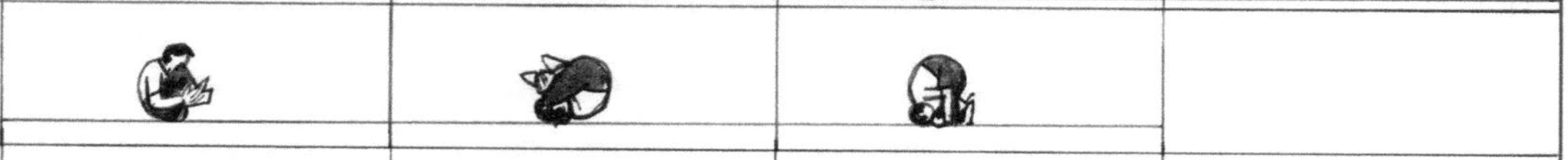
32 THE ROCKING	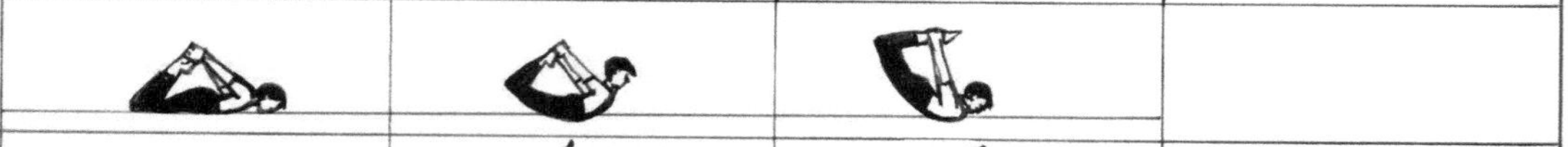
33 THE CONTROL BALANCE	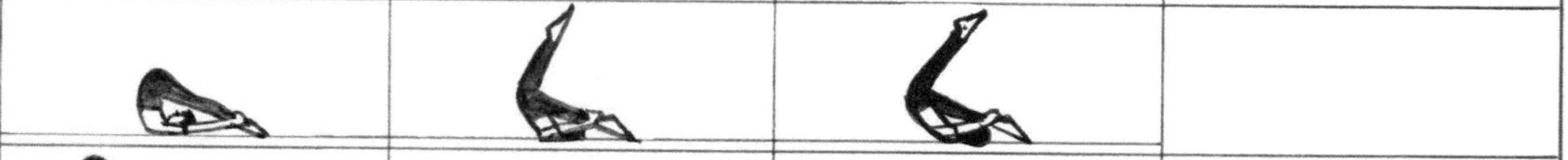
34 THE PUSH UP	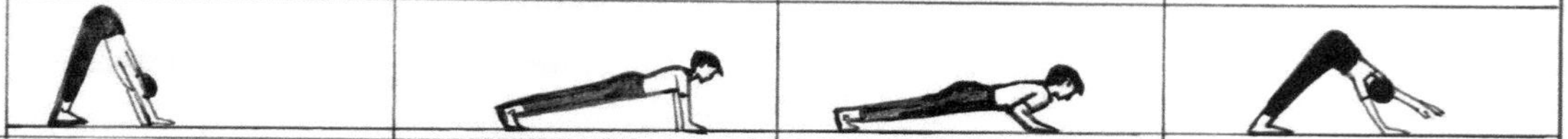

Conclusion

I hope you have enjoyed the previous pages and now have more of an understanding of Pilates. If you have managed to master some of the routines I hope you feel more flexible, fitter and stronger.

Above all I hope you have had fun.

My own experience of Pilates started with a bad back & a history of sports injuries but despite considering myself relatively fit I was astonished how hard it was to master even the tiniest movements. However I stuck with it & long dormant parts of my body started to wake up.

I am convinced that like me, there are many people who respond better to drawings than to words and whose imaginations are fired up by images. We are the visual-kinaesthetic learners who need to feel and see something to maximise our learning experience.

I am a Pilates teacher, have been a professional illustrator and am an unashamed doodler and comic enthusiast. In 2005 Suzanne Scott and I had the germ of an idea to make a book based on the teachings of the Scott Studio teacher training programme using my drawings and her knowledge. 12 years and many hours of teaching experience later, as well as long hours spent at the drawing board, a book was born. It encompasses The Scott Studio's desire to make Pilates accessible to as wide a group of people as possible, often modifying the original Pilates repertoire of 34 exercises whilst not losing their essential characteristics.

My job was to put pen to paper and make some pictures.

Acknowledgments

I would like to thank Jock and Suzanne Scott for their encouragement and endless work to raise the standards of movement education in the UK. Their energy and hard work is awe inspiring. Well respected teachers trained by this studio in Somerset can be found all over the world.

I am extremely grateful to the generous teachers who allowed me to use their classes in the book: Carla Barber, Liz Chandler, James D'Silva, Suzanne Scott, Liz Ellis and Carol Pirie. I love doing their classes!

Thank you to my initial readers Flick Baker, Joanna Briffa, Julia Cardozo, Yvonne Cash, Rob Dix, Phil Dobson, Liz Ellis, Nicky Holford, Diana Mowlam and Mike Hadley. You offered me unstinting advice and constructive criticism and without your time and help I would still be floundering.

To my clients past and present who inspire me every time I teach you. Without you this book would never have come into existence.

Resources

If you are looking for a well trained teacher, training courses or a Pilates studio try using these resources:

APPI Australian Physiotherapy and Pilates Institute: www.appihealthgroup.com

Balanced Body: www.pilates.com

Body Control Pilates: www.bodycontrolpilates.com

The Garuda Yoga and Pilates Studio: www.thegaruda.net

Independent Pilates Teachers Association: IPTA www.iptauk.com

Pilates Foundation: www.pilatesfoundation.com

The Scott Studio: info@thescottstudio.com

Stott Pilates: www.stott-pilates.co.uk

Pilates Anytime: www.pilatesanytime.com:
Online classes and courses taught by world class teachers

BV - #0022 - 140219 - C0 - 297/210/5 - PB - 9781910616819